Are Mental Disorders Brain Disorders?

The question of whether mental disorders are disorders of the brain has led to a long-running and controversial dispute within psychiatry, psychology and philosophy of mind and psychology. While recent work in neuroscience frequently tries to identify underlying brain dysfunction in mental disorders, detractors argue that labelling mental disorders as brain disorders is reductive and can result in harmful social effects.

This book brings a much-needed philosophical perspective to bear on this important question. Anneli Jefferson argues that while there is widespread agreement on paradigmatic cases of brain disorder such as brain cancer, Parkinson's or Alzheimer's dementia, there is far less clarity on what the general, defining characteristics of brain disorders are. She identifies influential notions of brain disorder and shows why these are problematic. On her own, alternative, account, what counts as dysfunctional at the level of the brain frequently depends on what counts as dysfunctional at the psychological level. On this notion of brain disorder, she argues, many of the consequences people often associate with the brain disorder label do not follow. She also explores the important practical question of how to deal with the fact that many people do draw unlicensed inferences about treatment, personal responsibility or etiology from the information that a condition is a brain disorder or involves brain dysfunction.

Anneli Jefferson is Lecturer in Philosophy, Cardiff University, UK. Her main research areas are moral philosophy and philosophy of psychology and psychiatry. She is especially interested in the intersection of these areas, for example in questions relating to moral psychology or the relationship between mental illness and moral responsibility.

Routledge Focus on Philosophy

Routledge Focus on Philosophy is an exciting and innovative new series, capturing and disseminating some of the best and most exciting new research in philosophy in short book form. Peer reviewed and at a maximum of fifty thousand words shorter than the typical research monograph, *Routledge Focus on Philosophy* titles are available in both ebook and print on demand format. Tackling big topics in a digestible format the series opens up important philosophical research for a wider audience, and as such is invaluable reading for the scholar, researcher and student seeking to keep their finger on the pulse of the discipline. The series also reflects the growing interdisciplinarity within philosophy and will be of interest to those in related disciplines across the humanities and social sciences.

Newton's Third Rule and the Experimental Argument for Universal Gravity
Mary Domski

The Philosophy and Psychology of Commitment
John Michael

The Ethics of Undercover Policing
Christopher Nathan

Are Mental Disorders Brain Disorders?
Anneli Jefferson

For more information about this series, please visit: www.routledge.com/Routledge-Focus-on-Philosophy/book-series/RFP

Are Mental Disorders Brain Disorders?

Anneli Jefferson

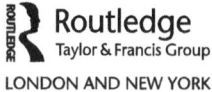
Routledge
Taylor & Francis Group

LONDON AND NEW YORK

First published 2022
by Routledge
4 Park Square, Milton Park, Abingdon, Oxon OX14 4RN

and by Routledge
605 Third Avenue, New York, NY 10158

Routledge is an imprint of the Taylor & Francis Group, an informa business

© 2022 Anneli Jefferson

British Library Cataloguing-in-Publication Data
A catalogue record for this book is available from the British Library

Library of Congress Cataloging-in-Publication Data
Names: Jefferson, Anneli, author.
Title: Are mental disorders brain disorders? / Anneli Jefferson.
Description: First edition. | Abingdon, Oxon ; New York, NY : Routledge,
[2022] | Series: Routledge focus on philosophy | Includes
bibliographical references and index.
Identifiers: LCCN 2022003172 (print) | LCCN 2022003173 (ebook) |
Subjects: LCSH: Brain—Diseases. | Neurobehavioral disorders.
Classification: LCC RC386 .J44 2022 (print) | LCC RC386 (ebook) |
DDC616.8—dc23/eng/20220224
LC record available at https://lccn.loc.gov/2022003172
LC ebook record available at https://lccn.loc.gov/2022003173

ISBN: 978-0-367-42138-0 (hbk)
ISBN: 978-1-032-30632-2 (pbk)
ISBN: 978-0-367-82208-8 (ebk)

DOI: 10.4324/9780367822088

Typeset in Bembo
by codeMantra

Contents

Acknowledgements

When I first started working on the philosophy of psychiatry, I was puzzled by how heated debates about whether mental disorders are brain disorders tend to be. This book is my attempt to untangle the debate and provide a workable notion of brain disorder applied to psychiatric conditions. Writing a book in a pandemic is not much fun, but the process has been greatly improved by the many people who have been generous with their time and comments. I have presented material from this book at Cardiff University, King's College London, the University of Wales Trinity Saint David, the Copenhagen 'Reactivity and Categorisations in the Human Sciences' Workshop and the BSPS and learned from my audiences and commentators. I would like to thank my colleagues in Cardiff for feedback on work in progress. I thank Nils Kürbis, Jon Webber and Katrina Sifferd for feedback on individual chapters. I was very fortunate to be able to workshop the manuscript with colleagues and friends, and thank Marko Jujarko, Luca Malatesti, Sofia Jeppsson, Sam Wilkinson, Marion Godman, Zsuzsanna Chappell, Liz Irvine, Tuomas Pernu and Harriet Fagerberg for their feedback. Special thanks go to David Papineau for support and incisive comments in this project and across the years, Jan-Hendrik Heinrichs for repeat reads and detailed feedback on everything, and Lisa Bortolotti for reading the whole manuscript and advising. I am also grateful to my two reviewers from Routledge for advice on how to further improve the manuscript and sharpen the presentation. Last but never least, I would like to thank my proof-reader extraordinaire and adviser on all things hardware-software distinction related, David Jefferson.

1 Introduction

1 The controversy surrounding 'brain disorder' labels

We often hear that specific mental health conditions are brain disorders or diseases. For example, the American Psychiatric Association characterizes schizophrenia as a chronic brain disorder (APA 2020). The authors of the Research Domain Criteria (RDoC), which is a system for classifying domains of psychological and brain function proposed by the United States' National Institute of Mental Health, also work on the assumption that mental disorders generally are brain disorders. We often hear statements like 'depression is a chemical imbalance in the brain'. At the same time, many scientists and philosophers strongly oppose characterizing conditions like depression, schizophrenia or bipolar as brain disorders. In a recent opinion piece in Nature, neuroscientist Carl Hart argued that categorizing addiction as a brain disease is both inaccurate and harmful to people suffering from addiction (Hart 2017). Psychologist Richard Bentall argues that viewing mental disorders as brain disorders gives us a skewed view of these conditions that does not take into account people's life history and the experiences that precipitated their mental distress.

We find ourselves in a strange stand-off: on the one hand, we have people saying that viewing mental disorders as brain disorders is the way forward in understanding and treating psychiatric conditions and applying this label will lead to more empathy towards people affected. On the other hand, many object that this view of psychiatric illness is both incorrect and harmful. According to both sides of the debate, there is a lot at stake in how we characterize these disorders, so we need to get this right.

Most people in the debate endorse a broadly materialist worldview, according to which mental processes depend on the brain, so

DOI: 10.4324/9780367822088-1

the disagreement does not rely on fundamentally different assumptions about the mind-brain relationship such as, for example, Cartesian dualism.[1] So why do researchers, clinicians and philosophers disagree so violently as to whether conditions such as addiction, schizophrenia, bipolar disorder or depression are brain disorders? In a recent piece defending the brain disorder view, neuroscientist Camilla Nord states: "I suspect the heart of the disagreement originates from people's vastly different ideas of what it means to say that something is a 'brain disorder'" (Nord 2021). This is the correct diagnosis, the main source of disagreement is a conceptual one, regarding the question what a brain disorder is. But, as with many stubborn disagreements, it isn't the case that we have clearly articulated conceptual differences – most of us aren't even sure what we mean by 'brain disorder', even if we have strong views on what *isn't* a brain disorder. While we agree about established cases of brain disorder such as neurosyphilis or Chorea Huntington, we lack good criteria for deciding how to categorize controversial cases such as addiction. Put differently, we may agree that a condition is a brain disorder when there is something wrong with the brain, but we don't agree on what differences from normal functioning count as there being something wrong with the brain.

The problem with discussions about brain disorders is that there are a number of ill-articulated presuppositions at play which lead to unhelpful confusion and disagreement. The two interconnected questions that will be running through this book are 'What is a brain disorder?' and 'What is the relationship between mental disorders and brain disorders?'. One important result from this book is that we have made so little progress on the second question because we don't have a clear answer to the first. So, I will propose criteria for dysfunction in the brain. On my account, mental disorders are brain disorders if they involve brain dysfunction, but they need not be caused by a preceding defect in the brain.

2 Methodology

Which mental disorders are brain disorders is an empirical question, but it requires a theory of what makes something a brain disorder. My aim is to answer this theoretical question. My approach to these issues is not an empirical but a philosophical one, clarifying the models that are used in the debate and their implications. The primary focus will be on what theoretical presuppositions underlie disagreements about brain disorders, and how these could be resolved. To illustrate the contrast to the empirical project, one could argue about whether addiction involves dopamine disregulation; this is an empirical question, and scientists need to look at the brains of healthy and addicted individuals to resolve it.

But often, the conceptual and the empirical are intermingled in these debates. We sometimes hear that bipolar disorder must be a brain disorder, because taking lithium helps to treat the symptoms. Or some say that depression cannot be a brain disorder because there is no single biological cause. These kinds of statements are of interest because of their hidden presuppositions. Working backwards from the claims made *about* brain disorders, I will tease out the presuppositions behind such claims and show what theories of brain disorder they commit people to. My own positive account will be theory driven, laying out conditions on when brain difference should count as brain dysfunction. Whether these conditions are met by mental disorders such as depression, schizophrenia or anorexia is, in the end, an empirical question. However, I will explain what kind of evidence and findings would support the claim that these conditions are brain disorders. Before embarking on the book's main argument, I will say a few words to explain what I mean by disorder and dysfunction, two key concepts in the book. I then distinguish my project from a related but slightly different discussion about the nature and benefits of the bio-psycho-social model of mental disorder versus the medical model.

3 Dysfunction and disorder

Much of this book will address the question of what a brain disorder is. But before addressing that in the main text, I want to briefly define the notions of mental disorder and of dysfunction, which are also central to these debates. People disagree about what mental disorders are and whether they exist in the first place; some feel they are better understood as problems in living. A further question is whether psychiatry even needs the concept of disorder in order to go about its business of treating people suffering from mental distress (Bortolotti 2020). I will not enter into these debates, but assume that we can make sense of the notion of mental disorder, even if there are borderline cases, where it will be hard to decide whether a condition should count as pathological. Dimensional approaches are increasingly popular in psychiatry, and if these are correct, the traits and symptoms that we have in extreme forms in conditions like schizophrenia, depression or obsessive compulsive disorder will often be present in less pronounced ways in the non-clinical population. So we should expect a certain amount of vagueness at the boundaries between health and illness.

I will be endorsing a hybrid account of mental disorder, according to which a mental disorder both requires psychological dysfunction and needs to meet a harmfulness criterion. In other words, I am not endorsing a purely naturalist account of mental disorder, which holds that mental disorders are conditions that do not require any normative judgements about desirability or rationality. (For a supposedly value-free account of mental disorder, see Christopher Boorse (1977).) Rather, I assume that in order to count as a disorder, a condition needs to be undesirable because it is harmful to the individual. While judgements of harm and desirability are frequently more controversial in the realm of mental health, we need to make these judgements even in the realm of somatic medicine. It may be more obvious that freedom from pain or a longer life expectancy are desirable, but we are still making an evaluative judgement when we say that they are.

Both dysfunction and harmfulness are necessary ingredients to an account of mental disorder: dysfunction is necessary, because not all disvalued and harmful states are considered disorders (so a harmfulness criterion cannot be sufficient). For example, Jerome Wakefield mentions the states of poverty and ignorance. Both are harmful to the individual, but they are not considered disorders (Wakefield 1992a). At the same time, not all psychological difference and not even everything described as psychological dysfunction is harmful to the individual or its environment, and harm is an essential part of our understanding of mental disorder.

3.1 Psychological difference/dysfunction

Physical or mental disorder requires dysfunction, whereby some organs or psychological processes in the agent are not operating as they are supposed to. As Wakefield has pointed out, this just raises the further question of how we decide what an organ, psychological mechanism, etc. are supposed to do (Wakefield 1992b). There are a number of options for addressing that particular gap, some of which aim to do more work than others. When is a difference in functioning a dysfunction? I take the broadest possible line here in order to avoid turf wars in the philosophy of medicine and biology. According to Robert Cummins (1975), we can define functions as contributions of a constituent part to the activity of a system it is embedded in. So, for example, the heart's function is to pump blood and this contributes to the transport of oxygen through the body. Other accounts of function define the function of an organ, trait or mechanism as its species-typical contribution to an organism's survival and reproduction (Boorse 1977) or as a selected effect (Wakefield 1992a, 2000, 2017b, Garson 2011, 2019).[2] What all these accounts have in common is that they think of function as a typical contribution of a trait/organ/mechanism to a larger scale goal or activity. Evolutionary or selected effect accounts of dysfunction think that we need to appeal to the effect a certain trait has had in the past which explains its retention in a population over generations. Many philosophers favour aetiological or evolutionary accounts of function partly because they think that this is what biologists mean by function (Garson 2019), but also because they provide a way of saying what something is good for without having to appeal to values. In this book, I will take dysfunction to be the failure of a trait or mechanism to contribute in the usual way to a system level capacity the organism has. Whether these contributions (functions) are selected for is a further question that I will remain agnostic about in this book.

3.2 Harmfulness

Both the notion of disorder and, to a lesser extent, that of dysfunction presuppose that there is something wrong with the agent. Unless one thinks that we can get the 'something wrong' out of evolutionary history, we will need to locate it in the fact that a condition is harmful to the person who has it. There are, of course, a bunch of thorny issues here, most prominently to what extent harm arises from the condition itself or from the way the social environment reacts and interacts with the person suffering from the condition. Famously, homosexuality is no longer considered a disorder because we came to the conclusion that in as far as homosexuality was harmful, this harm was caused by society's reaction to it, rather than by homosexuality itself. This means that our concrete diagnostic categories may need revision. (There are then further questions to be asked – whether it is sufficient for meeting that pre-condition if a mental health condition is typically, but not invariably, harmful to the individual (APA 2013, Cooper 2020).) While there are many tricky issues lurking in the background, in what follows, I will be assuming that mental disorders involve both psychological dysfunction and some form of harm.

4 Adjacent debates – the bio–psycho–social model and the medical model

The view that mental disorders are brain disorders is often equated with the medical model of mental disorder and contrasted with the bio–psycho–social model of mental disorder. On some readings, the medical model sees mental disorders as akin to somatic disorders and focuses on explanations and treatment methods that target the body, in the case of mental disorders, the brain. By contrast, psychotherapeutic approaches, heavily influenced by psychoanalysis, focus on psychology alone, and the bio-psycho-social model takes into account biological, psychological and social factors in its approach to mental illness (Roache 2020). Many authors now endorse the bio-psycho-social model for psychiatry (Bolton and Gillett 2019) and reject the medical model (though see Huda (2019) for a defence of the medical model that nevertheless acknowledges the importance of social and psychological factors).

While there is clearly an overlap between this debate and the issues I am interested in, my question is more narrow. My question is when we should say that there is something going wrong in the brain of someone suffering from a mental disorder that would justify speaking of a brain disorder. This is a much narrower focus, which is in principle compatible with different approaches to causal explanations for how someone got the condition in the first place and with different approaches to treatment. Furthermore, Engel's original proposal of the bio-psycho-social model stressed that we should take the psychological and social more seriously in both psychiatric *and* somatic conditions (Engel 1977). So it's not well suited to distinguish between different kinds of conditions. That biological and social factors should be attended to is a fairly well accepted point at this stage, as we know that things like low socio-economic status or loneliness are risk factors for somatic conditions as well and need to be considered in prevention and treatment (Huda 2019).

With these preliminaries in place, we can start tackling the main questions: what does it take to be a brain disorder; and can mental disorders be rightly labelled as brain disorders?

5 Outline of the argument

I will proceed as follows: in Chapter 2, I present and criticize one account of brain disorders that is prominent in the literature. On this narrow view of brain disorders, modelled on paradigmatic conditions such as neurosyphilis or brain tumours, mental disorders are indeed not brain disorders. However, as I will show, this account does not provide clear criteria for what it takes to be a brain disorder and so ends up being theoretically barren. When we say that depression is in many ways different from a classic brain disorder such as brain cancer or Parkinson's, we haven't said anything very informative. And the general criteria proposed either don't apply to all brain disorders or they are weak enough to be compatible with more modest accounts.

I then proceed to present my positive account in Chapter 3, which develops an account of mental disorders as brain disorders I first introduced in my paper "What does it take to be a brain disorder?" (Jefferson 2020b). On my account, a condition is a brain disorder if it is harmful and involves brain dysfunction. I define brain dysfunction as brain difference that realizes or causes psychological dysfunction. Much of the resistance to the brain disorder view stems from the fact that people ignore the possibility of dysfunctional *realizers* of mental dysfunction, focusing on preceding causes instead. In developing my own view, I also explain why a view according to which materialism implies that all mental disorders are *automatically* brain disorders is unsatisfactory and show that my theoretical approach fits nicely with the RDoC's understanding of mental disorders as brain disorders. (Though I am more agnostic than proponents of the RDoC about the question of whether we will actually be able to establish brain dysfunction for all mental disorders. Whether this is going to be possible depends on the extent to which we find systematic brain dysfunction in different mental disorders.)

In Chapter 4, I look at some common criticisms of brain disorder views and argue that while my view is reductionist in the sense that it requires explanatory reduction between the psychological and the brain level, this is not a problem. My account is not committed to another form of reduction which tries to explain psychiatric illness as resulting from one biological aetiology. I also address a further objection to views like mine, which is that biological psychiatry is internalist and locates dysfunction in the individual, whereas in reality, what counts as psychological dysfunction essentially depends on the external context. I concede a certain amount of context dependence, but defend a view of dysfunction that is internalist in important respects.

Finally, I address worries about the brain disorder view's implications for agency and responsibility in Chapter 5. We often hear that viewing a psychiatric illness as a brain disorder is stigmatizing and undermines the agency of individuals so diagnosed. After first probing and explaining the relationship between brain dysfunction and agency and responsibility, I address the prominent worries about labelling effects. Many argue that viewing mental disorders as brain disorders is detrimental to the people affected by the condition because of how it affects the way others and they themselves view them. A further concern holds that labelling a condition as a brain disorder leads to bad policy making. I investigate the empirical evidence for these claims and look at possible causes for these supposed negative effects and argue that, in as far as they exist at all, they rest on misunderstandings of the label and can be counteracted.

My hope is that this book can lay to rest many of the fruitless disagreements about brain disorders that we find both in the scientific literature and in popular media. A close analysis of what it means to say that a psychiatric illness involves dysfunction in the brain shows that the brain disorder label need not replace that of mental disorder and that we can acknowledge dysfunction in the brain without discounting the psychological perspective. Indeed, on my account we will often only be able to identify anomalies in brain processes as dysfunctional because they realize psychological dysfunction. In short, my aim is to mentalize the brain, rather than using the brain disorder label to discount the level of the mental.

Notes

1 I will explore the way in which beliefs about the mind–body relationship and views on the mental disorder/brain disorder relationship interact further in Chapter 3.
2 For an overview of different theories of function and their strengths and weaknesses when applied to psychiatric disorders, see Schramme (2010).

2 Brain disorders – the narrow view

1 Introduction

In this chapter, I argue that much of the strong resistance to the brain disorder view relies on a very specific notion of brain disorder which is modelled on infectious diseases such as syphilis. This view is attractive because it gives a unified account of the causes, symptoms and treatments of a disorder. However, it is theoretically underdeveloped because it is not specified how it can be extended beyond paradigm cases. I will call this account of brain disorders 'the narrow view', as it only counts conditions that closely resemble certain paradigmatic cases as brain disorders. I show how the narrow view has affected the debate and explain why it is an unsatisfactory notion of brain disorder. I will do so by looking at prominent objections to the view that mental disorders are brain disorders.

There is a prominent school of thought according to which mental disorders are not brain disorders because they are fundamentally different from paradigmatic brain disorders in a number of ways (Graham 2014, Pickard 2018, Borsboom, Cramer, and Kalis 2019). Frequently, this sharp distinction between mental disorders and brain disorders relies on the narrow view of brain disorders, which is at the same time overly demanding but also curiously underspecified. Analyzing the narrow view is informative, as it is one common way of understanding the term 'brain disorder' which drives rejection of the brain disorder label for mental health conditions. A further pay-off of this analysis is that it highlights the difficulties in finding criteria for calling a condition a brain disorder. Some readers may think the narrow view is a nonstarter as an account of brain disorders precisely because it is so narrow.[1] For those readers, this chapter can serve as an explanation of why some people object to the claim that mental disorders are brain disorders; and it can highlight some of the problems inherent in specifying what makes a condition a brain disorder.

DOI: 10.4324/9780367822088-2

The narrow view plays out in two ways in debates about mental disorders and brain disorders: one is the anti-psychiatry view, the view that mental disorders are not brain disorders, and hence, strictly speaking, not disorders at all. The other is the view that while mental disorders are genuine disorders, they are not brain disorders. The anti-psychiatry view was prominently defended by Thomas Szasz. While Szasz was himself a psychiatrist by training, he was also a leading figure in the anti-psychiatry movement. He put forward a definition of brain disorders according to which a condition is only a brain disorder if there is a defect in the brain which can be identified by biological science alone. Examples of such paradigmatic brain disorders are neurosyphilis, brain tumours, Parkinson's disease and Alzheimer's dementia. The most clear-cut case of a paradigmatic brain disorder is probably neurosyphilis, where mental symptoms are caused by bacterial infection. It is this underlying cause that needs treatment. More generally, the idea is that there should be an antecedent pathology in the brain, which can be treated by medication or surgery. I suspect that the prominence of these kinds of examples is one of the reasons that the term 'brain disease' is often used in preference to 'brain disorder'. While there is no commonly accepted distinction between brain disorders and diseases, the connotations are different. 'Brain disease' suggests some kind of organic failure, be this because of infection, cancer or insult to the brain. I will be using the term 'brain disorder', in analogy to 'mental disorder' in this book.[2]

Szasz argued that our understanding of illness and disease is fundamentally biomedical, and that mental disorders can only be understood as genuine disorders if they are brain disorders in the sense that there is some clearly identifiable brain defect that precedes psychological dysfunction and is identifiable by biomedical means alone. From this, he concluded that, as a matter of fact, mental disorders are not brain disorders in this strong sense. Instead, they are something altogether different, problems in living. It should, in fairness, be pointed out that Szasz took problems in living very seriously, and that denying that what we normally call mental disorders are genuine disorders was not meant to discredit the severity of the problems that people with conditions such as, for example, depression face.

Not everyone who denies that mental disorders are brain disorders is a sceptic about mental disorders or an anti-psychiatrist. Many psychologists, psychiatrists and philosophers argue that mental disorders are not brain disorders, but that they are nevertheless *bona fide* disorders. To a large extent, they endorse the narrow view espoused by anti-psychiatrists, as well as the belief that either all mental disorders are brain disorders or none of them are. Thus, while Szasz's and other anti-psychiatrists account of *mental* illness is rejected by most philosophers and clinicians, his characterization of *brain disorders* is endorsed by many authors who reject the view that mental disorders are brain disorders.

My aims in this chapter are the following:

1 Show that the belief that mental disorders are not brain disorders relies on a narrow and theoretically underspecified notion of brain disorders.

2 Explain why the idea that mental disorders are brain disorders in the narrow sense is attractive, but ultimately unhelpful.

3 Explore how the narrow view of brain disorders along with some assumptions about natural kinds can lead to the belief that either all mental disorders are brain disorders or none are.

4 Demonstrate that the notion of brain disorder employed both by anti-psychiatrists and those denying an overlap between mental disorders and brain disorders is theoretically underdeveloped. Developing and sharpening this distinction will likely lead to a broader notion which will include disorders over and above the paradigmatic cases normally appealed to in the discussion.

I will proceed as follows: first, I will outline the anti-psychiatry view that mental disorders are not brain disorders, and hence not proper disorders at all and the challenges it poses to psychiatry. I will then discuss the notion of brain disorder Szasz and many others hold and its problematic use of paradigm casts. Finally, I show how the understanding of brain disorders modelled on brain cancer, syphilis, etc. leads even some who accept the reality of mental disorders to reject the view that mental disorders are brain disorders. It will also become apparent that a further contributing factor to the dichotomy that many draw between mental disorders and brain disorders can be found in a common notion of natural kinds.

2 Anti-psychiatry and the view of brain disorders as 'real disorders'

Very few, if any, practitioners or philosophers endorse all of Szasz' views, and in particular, most authors reject his claim that mental disorders are only genuine disorders if they are also brain disorders (Banner 2013, Graham 2013a, Borsboom, Cramer, and Kalis 2019). Instead, they hold that mental disorders can be genuine disorders irrespective of whether there is any brain pathology involved. Nevertheless, parts of his view are still widely endorsed. Szasz's view of brain disorders as physiological or brain anatomical defects, which is modelled on paradigmatic conditions such as neurosyphilis or brain tumours, is widely shared by many philosophers and scientists. Plausibly, many authors have rejected Szasz' position regarding the relationship between mental disorders and brain disorders *because* they have bought into a definition of brain disorders much like the one Szasz endorses.

Szasz's account of brain disorders and the relationship between mental health conditions and brain disorders serves as an illustrative case study for a number of features of debates concerning the relationship between mental disorders and brain disorders.

1 Brain disorders are frequently defined in two complementary ways. The first is by ostension and analogy, where people say brain disorders are conditions which are like neurosyphilis, brain cancer, Parkinson's disease, etc. Some authors also give a seemingly clear-cut and well-defined definition of what it is to be a brain disorder. For example, according to Szasz, illness is defined as "the structural or functional alteration of cells, tissues and organs" (Szasz 2011, 179). This kind of definition operates in the tradition of the functional/organic distinction, which tries to subdivide disorders into organic conditions where we can find an underlying biological pathology (organic pathology) and those where this is not the case (Kendler 2012, Bell et al. 2020). We will see below that this notion of illness is ill-suited for describing psychiatric conditions.

2 One common assumption in the literature is that a pay-off of having a physiological criterion for categorizing a condition as a brain disorder is that it lends that condition scientific respectability. Being a brain disorder supposedly provides this respectability in two ways: first, it shows that mental disorders are not just disvalued states, but that there is something *physically* wrong with that person. We assume that in brain disorders, there is something wrong with a part of the body, the brain. Thus, the brain disorder label supposedly shows that there is something objectively wrong with us because our brain is broken. The second respectability worry concerns not the status of a mental health condition as a disorder, but whether classification picks out something that deserves to be labelled as a condition because it is sufficiently unified and distinct, ideally a natural kind. If scientists could find an underlying brain pathology, this would confirm the validity of diagnostic categories.

Diagnostic categories such as 'schizophrenia' or 'depression' are frequently criticized as not picking out genuine, separate conditions. Reasons for doubting diagnostic validity are (i) the heterogeneity of symptom clusters we find in different people with the same mental health diagnosis, and (ii) the fact that there are many overlapping symptoms between conditions and a lot of comorbidity. The worry is thus that whatever it is that psychiatrists are diagnosing when they diagnose a mental health condition, it is not a natural kind. Finding a biomarker, brain signature or whatever would seem to lend these diagnoses credibility if we could show that there are different brain anomalies in different psychiatric conditions.

3 Finally, Szasz and others explicitly draw some normative conclusions that many associate with the claim that mental disorders are brain disorders. For example, they argue that suffering from a brain disease exempts or excuses a person from moral and legal responsibility (Szasz 2011, Moncrieff 2020). If this was indeed a consequence, then establishing that a condition is a brain disorder would have important consequences beyond the purely medical. I will look at these normative issues in more detail in Chapter 5.

In his provocative landmark paper 'The myth of mental illness' (1960) Szasz claims that mental disorders are not, in fact, disorders at all, because they are not genuine forms of biomedical illness, as they do not involve pathology of the brain. So the two key claims Szasz makes are that (1) only disorders involving a breakdown of some sort in the body (including brain disorders like tumours or neurosyphilis) are genuine disorders; and that (2) mental disorders are not brain disorders.

As outlined above, most people working in the area of mental health reject this argument, because they reject the assumption that only conditions where there is pathology in the body can be disorders. Nevertheless, it is worth asking why people are drawn to the thought that mental disorders are only real disorders if we find a problem in the brain. Why the insistence on the importance of the physiological, on mental disorders being identifiable as disorders of the body? One obvious answer is that once we know what's gone wrong in the body, we can treat that problem. The relationship between disorder status and treatment method will be addressed in Section 3 of this chapter. But there are other motivations at play as well, which concern the status of mental disorders as genuine medical problems.

2.1   *The brain disorder label as a way of validating a condition as an illness*

One prominent motivation for saying that mental disorders are brain disorders (or hoping that they will be found to be) is that this will rehabilitate them as *bona fide* health conditions. Nomy Arpaly (2005) points out that positing that there is an 'imbalance in the brain' lends a mental disorder an air of tangibility and with that reality. The brain disorder label is thus well-suited to convince others of the reality and seriousness of the condition an individual is suffering from. (Though Arpaly believes that a well-established psychological diagnosis can have a similar, if weaker, effect.) We can also see this longing for a tangible, physical problem in reports of people dealing with mental illness or their relatives. A young man describes how the fact that there was no discernible physical illness made it harder for him to accept his mother's depression:

> There was something about not being able to see anything physically wrong with her that made me question whether it was really there at all.(...) I think the stigma surrounding mental health needs to be improved and it should be considered like any physical illness.
>
> (Rose 2017)

So far, I have described a psychological phenomenon, which is that mental disorders are taken more seriously as disorders if they are described as brain disorders. Possible explanations for this are that our understanding of mental disorders is modelled on somatic disorders, or that we think identifying brain pathology is the only way of differentiating between undesirable mental states and pathological ones. These thoughts certainly played an important role in the thinking of Szasz and the anti-psychiatry movement. However, the fact that calling something a brain disorder makes it seem more real is a psychological one. Something *seeming* more real does not yet imply that it *is* more real. Szasz, on the other hand, makes the much stronger claim that only somatic disorders – in this case, brain disorders – are real disorders.

It's worth noting that the idea that the only true (mental) disorders are brain disorders implies that people who suffer from conditions that cannot be categorized as brain disorders cannot in fact claim the disorder label for themselves. While this may be desirable for people who reject the idea that they are ill in the first place, we have seen that the disorder label performs a useful function for some people suffering from mental distress, by signalling that there is something objectively wrong with them and that they are not just 'acting up'. In as far as we accept the notion that only somatic (bodily) disorders are real disorders, we deprive people who are suffering from e.g. depression of a way of understanding themselves and being understood by others. This may be one of the reasons why we often get patients or relatives pushing the 'depression is a brain disorder' or 'addiction is a brain disorder' line.

However, in opposing the notion that conditions which are not somatic disorders are disorders, anti-psychiatrists see themselves as performing a service to people suffering from what we would ordinarily call mental illness. They fear that, absent some physiological criterion for illness, we end up evaluating other people's mental states as abnormal and pathological just because they deviate from some accepted societal norm: "what people now call mental illnesses are for the most part *communications* expressing unacceptable ideas, often framed, moreover, in an unusual idiom" (Szasz 1960, 116). So, one driving idea in Szasz's account and that of other critics of psychiatry is the belief that calling a condition a mental disorder unjustifiably pathologizes problems in living.

Most people would agree that mere unhappiness or deviation from social norms is insufficient for the diagnosis of a mental illness. It is also a matter of regrettable historical fact that psychiatry has been misused in the past to pathologize behaviour that was inconvenient for those in power. One example is 'sluggish schizophrenia', a disorder diagnosed in dissidents in the Soviet Union (Wilkinson 1986). In fact, avoiding this kind of abuse of mental health diagnoses is an explicit goal in recent versions of the Diagnostic and Statistical Manual of Mental Disorders. The DSM5 states: "Socially deviant behavior (e.g. political, religious, or sexual) and conflicts that are primarily between the individual and society are not mental disorders unless the deviance or conflict results from a dysfunction in the individual" (APA 2013, 20).

Given the troubled history of mental health diagnoses, it is understandable that psychiatry wants to find a way of avoiding the accusation that our mental health categories are just ways of pathologizing psychological difference. One way of doing this would be to show that mental disorder diagnoses are value free. But, as I state in the introduction, medicine is not value free and psychiatric diagnosis need not be completely value free. There are plenty of hybrid accounts which hold that there is both a clearly delineable condition with psychological states that deviate from normal functioning and an evaluative, normative element (Cooper 2020). For example, Wakefield argues for an account that defines dysfunction in terms of evolutionary theory, as a failure of an organ or mechanism to perform the function it was evolved to perform, but also requires that the condition should be harmful for the individual or their environment (Wakefield 2017a, 1992b). Furthermore, somatic medicine itself is not value free. So, while the issue of values poses more of a problem for psychiatry than it does for somatic medicine, this is a difference in degree, not in kind.

3 How the narrow view defines brain disorders

While they disagree on the reality of mental disorder, anti-psychiatrists like Szasz and many psychologists, psychiatrists and philosophers who defend the reality of mental illness agree that mental disorders are not brain disorders. This is not because they disagree with the view that all mental states require brain states for their existence, or because they reject the idea that brain science can teach us about the mind. In order to find out why they object to the brain disorder label being applied to mental illness, we need to look more closely at what they mean by 'brain disorder'. Obviously, not everyone who says that mental disorders are not brain disorders has a clear idea of what a brain disorder is. But they need to have at least a vague notion that allows them to say that mental disorders aren't like 'that'. The main motivation for saying that mental disorders are not brain disorders appears to be the thought that in most mental health conditions, there is no clearly identifiable brain pathology. But that does not help, as it just replaces the question what a brain disorder is with the one what clearly identifiable brain pathology is.

To figure out what people mean by 'brain disorder' it may be useful to look at cases everybody agrees are brain disorders. In some disorders that are associated with mental health symptoms, finding biological causes that affect the brain has led to a medical breakthrough in understanding and treating the condition. For example, patients suffering from disorders like syphilis or Chorea Huntington have mental symptoms that can also be found in conditions like depression or schizophrenia, but these can be explained by a bacterial infection or genetic defect. So, one understanding of mental disorders as brain disorders is that they are conditions like syphilis, where finding brain pathology would give us the key to the aetiology and treatment of the condition. Jennifer Radden elegantly summarizes this model of mental disorders as brain disorders which have a single underlying cause.

> For each distinct disease, a single, specific, cellular-level cause must be sought (Virchow), when any such finding requires independent verification (Koch). Together, these principles, expectations, and demands, laid out a model or picture of disease ontology comprising

an underlying core causally responsible for its more readily observable signs and symptoms which, as downstream effects, provided clues to the real, underlying disease entity or process.

(Radden 2018, 1088)

The thought that mental disorders might be explained in this way is attractive both theoretically and in terms of treatment options. As Ian Hacking points out, finding out the cause of a condition helps explain it, prevent it and cure it, but more than that, it reassures us that we have "identified a disease entity, something more than a cluster of symptoms" (Hacking 1995, 81). However, psychiatrists generally no longer believe that this model can be applied to most mental disorders (Kendler 2005, Walter 2013). Rather, current biological psychiatry aims to discover realizers of mental symptoms in the brain, thus adding to our understanding of the condition and possible ways of treatment.

Nevertheless, cases like syphilis clearly shape Szasz's concept of brain disorders: he envisions brain disorders to be conditions which have a physical cause which leads to mental symptoms, and can be treated by interventions on the body. Here is Szasz on the topic of what makes something a brain disorder (or 'disease' in his terminology):

The crux of the matter is that a disease of the brain, analogous to a disease of the skin or bone, is a neurological defect, and not a problem in living. For example, a *defect* in a person's visual field may be satisfactorily explained by correlating it with certain *definite lesions* in the *nervous* system.

(Szasz 1960, 113)

Szasz's primary examples of brain pathology are lesions, structural defects in the brain, often due to injury. His general characterization of brain disorders defines them as "the structural or functional alteration of cells, tissues and organs" (Szasz 2011, 179).

When structural alterations in the brain result from injury, it is straightforward to say that there is damage to the brain. However, not all structural or functional deviations from the norm are pathological. The class of functional alterations of the brain includes a host of different kinds of cases. For example, in a famous study researchers found that London cab drivers had increased volume in their hippocampus (Maguire et al. 2000); this structural change merely reflects the brain's reaction to the cognitive demands of being a cab driver on spatial memory. So, both for structural and functional alterations in the brain, we need a way of defining dysfunction. Just how difficult that can be is brought out by a recent criticism of autism research by Laurent Mottron, who points out that "variations in cortical volume have been ascribed to a deficit when they appear in autism, regardless of whether the cortex is thicker or thinner than expected" (Mottron 2011, 34). Thus, we need an understanding of brain processes and psychological processes (and whether these are dysfunctional) to establish which alterations in the brain are dysfunctional. Positing the existence of dysfunction for a condition being a brain disorder does not specify how we define dysfunction on the level of the brain and is therefore in need of further specification.

One might think that there is an easy response here; we could say that any brain differences that underlie psychological dysfunction are therefore brain dysfunctions, so that we are dealing with brain disorders in these cases. Indeed, I will defend a view along those lines in Chapter 3. But proponents of the narrow view reject this solution. George Graham, for example, explicitly resists the idea of defining brain disorders as brain anomalies that realize psychological dysfunction. Rather, the idea seems to be that we can have a standard of brain dysfunction that is independent of, and prior to, that of mental dysfunction.

> The identity of a mental with a neural disorder (…) is supposed to mean that the very ideas of a neural disorder and of how the brain is supposed to operate if healthy, properly regimented or explicated, should be used to explain what makes something a mental disorder.
> (Graham 2013a, 24).

So the notion of brain pathology is supposed to be prior to, even independent of, mental dysfunction.

As a way of fleshing out their view, Szasz and many other authors provide a general definition like the one cited above and then give examples of the kind of conditions they have in mind. In the literature, we find a recurring list of paradigmatic cases of brain disorders associated with mental symptoms: neurosyphilis, brain tumours, delirious conditions such as those brought about by intoxicants and thiamine deficiency (Szasz 1960, 2011, Walter 2013, Pickard 2018). However, paradigmatic examples are not enough to decide the extension of the term 'brain disorder'. In effect, what listing paradigmatic examples does is to point the finger at a group of diseases and tell us 'something like that is a brain disease'. But it does not provide any way of moving beyond paradigm cases and adjudicating controversial ones. One strategy for progressing beyond paradigmatic cases when deciding what falls under the extension of the term 'brain disorder' is ostension and analogy: one can posit that diseases which are *like* brain tumours or neurosyphilis are brain disorders.

However, even if we proceed by analogy, we will need to spell out *what* similarities to paradigmatic cases matter. We can then proceed by comparing a condition to a paradigmatic brain disorder. One of the features of that paradigmatic brain disorder can then be proposed as a condition for category membership.[3] So we get arguments for category membership along the following lines:

Condition *x* is a brain disorder because it is like paradigmatic brain disorder *y* in respect *p*.

Or, alternatively:

Condition *x* is not a brain disorder because it is unlike paradigmatic brain disorder in respect *p*.

The corresponding definition of a brain disorder would then be:

A condition is a brain disorder *iff* it is like paradigmatic brain disorders in respect *p*.

We can see this pattern of establishing membership in the category 'brain disorder' at work in objections to the view that addiction is a brain disorder. For example, in a piece by Sally Satel and Scott Lilienfield from 2017, the comparison to paradigmatic brain diseases is used to show how addiction differs from classic brain disorders in important respects. This difference is then used to establish that addiction is *not* a brain disorder. Satel and Lilienfeld criticize Michael Boticelli, who was President Obama's drug czar, for drawing the analogy between brain cancer and addiction. Boticelli claimed that just like cancer, addiction is a disorder of the body, in this case, the brain. They quote him as saying "We don't expect people with cancer to stop having cancer" and then go on to say:

> Botticelli's analogy doesn't work. No amount of reward or punishment can alter the course of, say, brain cancer. It is an entirely autonomous biological condition. Imagine threatening to impose a penalty on a brain cancer victim if her vision or speech continued to worsen or to offer (…) $1 million if she could stay well. It wouldn't matter.(…) The brain disease model also fosters an unrealistic medication campaign.
>
> (Satel and Lilienfeld 2017)

There is a lot going on in this quote, but what I want to draw attention to is the pattern of reasoning we find, implicitly or explicitly, in a lot of writing on the mental disorder/brain disorder distinction.

P1: Only those conditions which can be treated by biological intervention are (paradigmatic) brain disorders.

P2: Mental disorders like addiction respond to psychological interventions.
C: Therefore, mental disorders like addiction are not brain disorders.

In essence, one prominent feature of paradigmatic brain disorders has been made into a necessary criterion for being a brain disorder; it has been made definitional. We find a similar line of thought in Szasz, whose narrow view only counts conditions that can be treated through surgery or medication and who insists that brain pathology has to causally precede any mental symptoms.

Clearly, not all features of paradigmatic brain disorders are suitable candidate conditions for category membership. At the very least, they need to be shared between paradigmatic cases. For example, syphilis is a bacterial infection, whereas Alzheimer's, Parkinson's and other paradigmatic conditions are not. So being a bacterial infection can't be a necessary condition for being a brain disorder. A decision on what features matter is essential to resolving debates on whether a condition is a brain disorder. Otherwise people end up talking past each other. Here is an example of how this can happen: in an opinion piece, Carl Hart argues against the brain disorder view of addiction (partly) on the basis that paradigmatic brain disorders are progressive and irreversible without medical treatment, whereas addiction is not (Hart 2017). In a response to Hart's paper, Bedi et al. use the same argumentative strategy of drawing an analogy to paradigmatic disorders and stress that "neuroimaging studies have shown that neurobiological function in SUDs (substance use disorders) differs markedly from healthy individuals and these differences can have comparable size effects to those in diseases like Huntingdon's or Parkinson's" (Bedi et al. 2017).

What these kinds of disagreements show us is that the approach of extracting criteria for category membership by looking at common features of paradigm cases (a) relies on there being such shared features, and (b) that these features are suitable for deciding category membership. A shared feature that is, as it were, incidental will not provide a good candidate criterion for membership in the category 'brain disorder'. The most prominent criteria for membership in the category 'brain disorder' we find in the literature are aetiology or (and this is an inclusive or) treatment method. These two come up time and again in the literature; we have already seen that Satel and Lilienfeld appeal to the latter: treatment.

Hanna Pickard's take on the mental disorders as brain disorders view illustrates appeal to both these criteria.

The hope of biological psychiatry is that we will ultimately discover an underlying brain pathology that is the common cause of the psychological and behavioural symptoms diagnostic of each type of mental disorder, just as we have discovered specific physical pathologies that underlie the surface symptoms of many physical diseases. But despite great advances in the cognitive and neurobiological sciences and much research dedicated to this hope, at most twice in the history of psychiatry has this model proven apt. Around the turn of the 20th C, scientists discovered that, in some patients, the collection of symptoms of paranoia, grandiosity, and confusion, was caused by tertiary syphilis, which can be treated with antibiotics. More than one hundred years later, preliminary studies conducted over the last few years have suggested that other cases of first-time psychosis may be caused by specific antibodies in the blood, which respond to immunotherapy.

(Pickard 2018)

I will consider aetiology and treatment in turn.

Aetiology: the aetiological criterion holds that the causal explanation for the disorder should make reference to dysfunction in the brain. Intuitively, the causal story goes something like this: first your brain breaks, then your psychology follows suit. Pickard's example of syphilis illustrates this nicely. A bacterial infection is what damages the brain, and that is what leads to mental symptoms. This way of thinking is reflected in the functional/organic distinction in psychiatry. As attractive as it is, the model of bacterial infection that we have in neurosyphilis where we have one clear cause does not apply to a number of other conditions, be they somatic or psychiatric. The causes of mental disorders are multiple and varied, as has been prominently argued by Kendler (2012). Furthermore, and importantly, the causes of a number of bodily diseases are also multiple and varied, and include psychological factors such as stress (Bolton and Gillett 2019) for heart disease. Bacterial and viral infections only form a very small subset of health conditions. Given the multiple risk factors we have even for somatic disorders, the idea that all brain disorders should only have one cause seems like a non-starter.

Another possible claim thinkers like Pickard might be making is that even if we allow for multiple risks and 'difference makers' we are only dealing with a brain disorder if it's the case that first the brain breaks, then the mind does as a result. In the case of neurosyphilis, bacterial infection causes the brain to break. But you might be happy to concede that stress could be a contributing factor to a brain defect while still holding that the problem in the brain precedes and explains the mental health problem. (So, to use a hypothetical example, if it were the case that stress was a contributing factor to brain cancer, we could admit that psychological factors can lead to brain disorder, while at the same time insisting that any psychological symptoms (for example disinhibition) resulting from the tumour should be explained as a result of the changes in the brain.) We find a similar assumption that we can trace certain mental symptoms to pathology in the brain in the functional/organic distinction, which subdivides conditions into organic ones where we can find a biological cause and functional ones where this is not the case. However, Bell et al. (2020) argue that the functional/organic distinction as a distinction between causes for mental symptoms is neither well-conceived nor consistently adhered to in psychiatry. It also does not clearly classify along the same lines as the mental disorder/ brain disorder distinction, if we allow functional brain anomalies into the set of things that can constitute brain pathology.

The narrow view, according to which all the aetiological and explanatory action needs to be located at the level of the brain, does not leave much space for mental disorders to be brain disorders. But, as we have seen, it is a picture that only describes a small subset of conditions, be they somatic or psychiatric, in the first place. The conclusion that because most conditions aren't like syphilis, they can't be brain disorders, only follows if we insist that the brain needs to be the exclusive locus of causal, purely mechanistic explanation.

What about focusing on treatment methods in order to decide whether a condition is a brain disorder? This is a very prominent idea in Szasz's work, and it is also one of the factors that motivated biological psychiatry in the second half of the 20th century. Anecdotally, it is also a common factor people appeal to in defending the claim that a certain condition is a brain disorder. For example, a neuroscientist once told me that "Of course bipolar disorder is a brain disorder, it responds to lithium." There are two ways of understanding the claim that being treatable by medication, surgery or some other direct physical intervention on the brain makes a condition a brain disorder. The first is to interpret the success of a treatment method as evidential. If the correct path of intervention is via physical intervention on the brain, then the problem must also lie in the brain. So, rather than being a criterion in its own right, the method of intervention provides evidence for the claim that we are dealing with brain dysfunction.

This evidential claim is of course fallible, as a recent discussion of serotonin reuptake inhibitors shows. Lacasse and Leo criticize the move from the claim that SSRIs (serotonin reuptake inhibitors) are successful in some patients to the one that this supports the hypothesis that depression results from a serotonin deficit.

> [T]he claimed efficacy of SSRIs is often cited as indirect support for the serotonin hypothesis. Yet, this *ex juvantibus* line of reasoning (i.e., reasoning "backwards" to make assumptions about disease *causation* based on the response of the disease to a *treatment*) is logically problematic—the fact that aspirin cures headaches does not prove that headaches are due to low levels of aspirin in the brain.
>
> (Lacasse and Leo 2005, 1212)

So the evidential claim is merely that: evidential. In order to do more than provide potential evidence for brain pathology, we need to posit a disease mechanism that we can clearly characterize as a case of brain pathology. Ideally, the success of treatment would lend support to the postulated underlying dysfunction, but it would not replace such a notion of dysfunction.

The second option is to move directly from the claim that a disorder is treated via physiological intervention on the brain to the conclusion that it is a brain disorder. This is, in essence, a pragmatic way of categorizing disorders. Rather than worrying about where to locate the dysfunction, we just classify by practice. If it's treated by medication, then it's a brain disorder. If it's treated by talking therapy, it's a mental disorder. This is not a ridiculous way of proceeding. Medicine is, after all, just as much a practical endeavour as it is a science. However, there are paradigmatic brain disorders which do not require direct treatment of the brain. For example, while acute stroke is treated through medication, the after-effects of stroke are treated through physical and speech therapy, rather than through direct intervention on the brain. Furthermore, treatment of many psychiatric conditions is not either purely physiological or purely aimed at the mind. We are, once again, in a different situation to the one we find ourselves in as regards neurosyphilis, where antibiotics are the silver bullet. Treatment of mental health conditions normally makes use of different interventions. Psychiatrists can use both medication and psychological treatment. Bipolar disorder, for example, is frequently treated through both medication and psychotherapeutic approaches.

The reality is that treatment of mental illness does not fit with the dichotomy between mental disorders and brain disorders. If the criterion for being a brain disorder is therefore that psychopharmaceutical treatment (or electro-convulsive therapy, or surgery) should be the only treatment, then the set of brain disorders is unlikely to change significantly from the paradigmatic cases we are already familiar with. If we insist that only those conditions treated by direct physical interventions are brain disorders, this will restrict the set of brain disorders to those kinds of conditions we already label as paradigmatic brain disorders, even if we take treatment to be purely pragmatic criterion. It is of course possible that a number of further conditions might be added in future, assuming there is a medical breakthrough that finds a hitherto unknown one-stop treatment for specific mental health conditions. Alternatively, those conditions which respond to different and combined treatment approaches would naturally be classified as both mental and brain disorders. This is incompatible with the dichotomy between mental disorders and brain disorders, but if we give up this dichotomy, we can hold that a condition is both a mental disorder and a brain disorder.[4]

The idea that there is a clearly delineable set of brain disorders runs into the problem of specifying when the brain counts as diseased. Common responses to this question tend to highlight either the aetiology of a condition or the way it is treated. However, we have seen that both aetiology and treatment are normally multi-factorial. If we think that clearly definable and identifiable damage in the brain needs to precede mental symptoms and that treatment needs to directly intervene on the brain and fix the identified dysfunction in the brain, there will be very few brain disorders. Furthermore, and more importantly, we have not been given any principled reason to say that those conditions where we do have clear brain differences, even if there are psychological risk factors and treatment options, should *not* count as brain disorders.

4 Beyond Szasz – the narrow view of brain disorders in current debates

While Szasz's restrictive position on brain disorders is not well motivated, many philosophers, psychologists and (to a lesser extent) psychiatrists agree with Szasz that mental disorders are not brain disorders; and many endorse a view of brain disorders similar to that of Szasz. However, the majority of mental health professionals and philosophers of medicine reject Szasz's claim that there are no mental disorders. Rather, they have developed accounts that stress the autonomy of mental illness. In doing so, they have been too willing to accept the divide between 'proper brain disorders' and other conditions. In many instances, philosophers have replaced Szasz' dichotomy between brain disorders and problems of living with a trichotomy between brain disorders, mental disorders and problems in living. For example, George Graham argues that bipolar disorder can be either a mental disorder or a brain disorder, but not both, and if we found out it was definitely a brain disorder, that would "force [it] off of the list" of mental disorders on to that of brain disorders (Graham 2013a, 38).

One motivation why thinkers like Graham insist that mental disorders can't be brain disorders, already outlined above, is simply that they endorse the narrow view of brain disorders. Another possible justification for this way of carving up the conceptual landscape may be the assumption that types of disorders form natural kinds. If natural kind categories cut nature at its joints, then, on many conceptions of natural kinds, they should not overlap (Cooper 2013, Bird and Tobin 2018). But, unless we commit ourselves to the claim that mental disorders and brain disorders are natural kinds like gold and silver, different and wholly distinct at a parallel level of classification, there is no reason to believe that there cannot be any overlap between the categories. On a very naive reading, we might think that the way we think about chemical elements is a natural way of thinking about mental disorders and brain disorders, too, as they are different kinds of medical conditions. But this would be inaccurate. Irrespective of what we end up saying about the relationship between mental disorders and brain disorders, it's pretty clear that mental disorders rely on the brain, just as all other mental states do. So taking chemical elements as a model does not work. Disorder categories which are at the intersection of a number of special sciences are not noticeably similar to chemical elements. The chemical elements account of natural kinds is of course not the only way of understanding natural kinds. I am merely presenting it as a possible explanation for why we sometimes find the assumption that mental disorders and brain disorders are dichotomous.

5 Conclusion

In this chapter, I have introduced and criticized a restrictive notion of brain disorders. Authors who hold this kind of view have argued that mental disorders are not brain disorders. They have taken this to show (a) either that there are no mental disorders at all or (b) that the categories of mental disorder and brain disorder are completely distinct. The two most frequently encountered criteria people use to establish whether a condition is a brain disorder are aetiology and treatment. However, both the aetiology and the treatment of mental disorders normally involve physiological *and* psychological processes. This means that a picture that insists on an all-or-nothing role for the brain in order to categorize a condition as a brain disorder will indeed not categorize conditions such as schizophrenia or bipolar disorder as brain disorders. But this is a result of defining dysfunction at the level of the brain in an extremely narrow way. There is nothing in the notion of dysfunction itself that says that an anomaly in the brain (be it structural or functional) can only count as brain dysfunction if it fulfils the same causal and explanatory role as it does in paradigmatic brain disorders. While the narrow view ends up not being satisfactory, it has a strong appeal: first of all, it aims to tell a causal story where pathology in the brain precedes mental symptoms and it is this very pathology that must be addressed directly (not via therapy) in order to cure the patient. It tries to align brain disorders with somatic medicine more generally and with its insistence that we need to be able to point to specific dysfunction in the brain in order to say that we are dealing with a brain disorder. The vexed question is just how to establish that there is such dysfunction.

Notes

1 In fact, I have been confronted with the objection that 'nobody really holds this view'. I find this objection rather baffling, as there are a number of people I cite in this chapter who clearly endorse this view of brain disorders and consequently reject the view that mental disorders are brain disorders. Furthermore, it is in many ways an attractive view in the way it unifies all explanation at the level of the brain, so it is by no means a strawman position. The unfortunate reality is just that it presupposes a unified causal pathway that we do not find in actual mental disorders.

2 A further common distinction in the literature is that between disorder or disease and illness. But once again, this is not used consistently across the literature. Some authors use it to distinguish between all pathological conditions (disorder/disease) and those that require medical attention (illness) (Boorse 1975); others use the term 'illness' to refer to the lived experience and phenomenology of the condition (Boyd 2000). I will not be using the term 'illness' in any theoretically loaded way.

3 One might object that the appeal to paradigm cases lends itself to a rather different understanding of brain disorders, where the boundary between conditions that are brain disorders and those that aren't is fuzzy. This would be more in keeping with the prototype theory of concepts (Margolis and Laurence 2021), which does not posit necessary and sufficient conditions for concept membership. I am sympathetic to this objection. Nevertheless, I will put it to one side for now, because this is clearly not the way appeal to paradigm cases works in the literature, where it is used as a criterion for exclusion or inclusion.

4 One might also object that even this way of distinguishing between treatment of the brain and treatment of the mind is misguided because psychological treatment, like all our experiences, affects the brain. I am sympathetic to this objection, but we have seen in the quotes that there is at least an intuitive distinction between, as it were, intervening directly on the hardware as a form of treatment and making changes via mental processes. If one doesn't accept this intuitive distinction between interventions on the brain that are purely medical or mechanical and mental interventions, then the narrow notion of brain disorders will seem unappealing from the get-go.

3 A workable notion of brain dysfunction

1 Introduction

We have seen that there is agreement that brain disorders require brain dysfunction, but that there is no agreement on what makes a brain process, structure or state dysfunctional. On the strong notion of brain disorder, it is indeed incorrect to say that mental disorders are brain disorders. On these accounts, only lesions such as those we find in paradigmatic brain disorders count as brain pathology and can underwrite the term 'brain disorder'. Putative defining criteria for brain dysfunction, such as aetiology and treatment, are not well-suited to separate 'genuine' brain disorders from other conditions that involve the brain, particularly conditions such as bipolar disorder or schizophrenia, in which both pharmaceutical and psychological treatment plays an important role. Of course, there is a difference between paradigmatic brain disorders such as brain cancer and conditions such as depression. Psychological treatment plays a central role in the latter in a way that it doesn't in the former. Nevertheless, even in the case of depression, there will be cases where treatment primarily targets the brain, either in the form of medication or, more controversially, Electro-Convulsive Therapy.

Aetiological or causal explanation and treatment do not yield clear boundaries between brain disorders and mental disorders. Furthermore, while a preceding cause of psychological symptoms is a good candidate criterion for making a brain anomaly a dysfunction, this does not mean that an anomalous brain process that realizes a psychological dysfunction should not count as disordered. Indeed, many psychiatrists and philosophers take a different approach and argue that physicalism in and of itself implies that all mental disorders are brain disorders. Proponents of biological psychiatry also hold that we should reject Cartesian Dualism (Kendler 2005), according to which there are two distinct substances, mind (*res cogitans*) and matter (*res extensa*), which exist

DOI: 10.4324/9780367822088-3

independently of each other and interact. Rather, biological psychiatrists endorse physicalism; the thesis that matter is the only real stuff
that there is. Physicalism is thought to be the theory that is supported by
"an overwhelming degree of clinical and scientific evidence" (Kendler
2005, 434).

However, the belief that biological psychiatry is incompatible with
physicalism or that physicalism entails that all mental disorders are brain
disorders ignores some theoretical options in the philosophy of mind.
Conversely, claiming that physicalism entails that all mental disorders
are brain disorders is too hasty. My own view is physicalist, but I will
nevertheless briefly consider the implications dualism has for biological
psychiatry. In the following sections, I show that the assumption that
biological psychiatry is incompatible with dualism is only true for certain types of dualism; and that the claim that physicalism necessarily
implies that all mental disorders are brain disorders is incorrect. After
establishing this, I put forward my positive proposal, which spells out
brain dysfunction as brain difference that causes or realizes psychological dysfunction. I call this the inclusive view of brain disorders. As
I will argue, realization of psychological dysfunction is sufficient for
brain dysfunction. The brain dysfunction need not also have temporally
preceded and caused the psychological dysfunction. Finally, I will show
that my account makes good sense of the way proponents of the RDoC
conceptualize mental disorders as brain disorders.

2 The mind-body relationship and its implications for psychiatry

2.1 Biological psychiatry and dualism

In this book I won't defend either dualism or physicalism, though I
myself am a physicalist. Nevertheless, it's worth showing that not all
forms of dualism are incompatible with biological psychiatry and the
view that mental disorders are brain disorders. It is true that an extreme
form of dualism, according to which mind and brain act largely independently, is hard to square with biological psychiatry and neuroscience
more generally.[1]

But there are other forms of dualism, which take the mental to be
irreducibly subjective and therefore separate from the physical that do
not engender these kinds of problems. Even if we are reductionists
about the explanation of mental illness to the extent that we think that
all psychological *mechanisms* can be given a brain explanation, Maung
(2019) argues that there are other types of dualism such as Chalmers's

naturalist dualism – a form of property dualism – which are compatible with the reductionist project in psychiatry. Chalmers's style dualism would allow for the reduction of cognitive processes, but not of the phenomenal quality of mental *states*. Chalmers is a dualist because he believes that phenomenal character of mental states, the 'what it is like' of feeling sad, enjoying the taste of chocolate or experiencing a thought insertion are not reducible to the physical and that therefore, the mental is different from the physical. Nevertheless, *psychological processes* are, at least in principle, reducible and these are the ones that biological psychiatry seeks to explain.

> [Chalmers'] variety of dualism contends that first-person subjective experience is a further fact that is numerically and metaphysically distinct from the physical facts, but fully accepts that it is nomologically related to physical processes and that the psychological processes involved in the causation of behaviour are explainable in terms of such physical processes in a biological system. This is entirely compatible with the biological psychiatry thesis that psychiatric disorders are grounded in biological processes. Hence, we can accept that this variety of dualism is true while taking seriously the scientific claims of biological psychiatry.
>
> (Maung 2019, 68)

In summary, while there is widespread rejection of dualism among psychiatrists, biological psychiatry is in principle compatible at least with a modest property dualism of the Chalmers kind, as is the claim that mental disorders might be brain disorders. So, as a blanket claim, the assertion that dualism precludes biological psychiatry and the option that mental disorders are brain disorders are incorrect. Conversely, this also means that you cannot just infer physicalism from an endorsement of biological psychiatry. There's no simple series of implications from 'biological psychiatry' to 'physicalism'. Thus, some forms of dualism are still on the table. Now I will argue that even if we endorse physicalism, there is no automatic entailment relation between 'physicalism is true' and 'all mental disorders are brain disorders'.

2.2 Does physicalism imply that all mental disorders are brain disorders?

We have seen that biological psychiatry need not endorse physicalism and that even if we were to accept a modest dualism, there would still be scope for mental disorders to be brain disorders. But many psychiatrists do explicitly commit themselves to physicalism, and this is also the most commonly defended position in philosophy.

What implications does accepting physicalism have for the relationship between mental disorders and brain disorders? Kendler claims that "The rejection of Cartesian dualism logically leads to the conclusion that all psychiatric disorders are biological" (Kendler 2005, 434). Saying that all psychiatric disorders are biological is not exactly the same as saying that all mental disorders are brain disorders, but one can move from one claim to the other in a few short steps:

P1   All psychiatric disorders are biological disorders.
P2   Biological disorders involve some problem with the body.
P3   The brain is the part of the body implicated in psychiatric disorders.
C1   All psychiatric disorders involve some problem in the brain.
P5   All disorders that involve some problem in the brain are brain disorders.
C2   All psychiatric disorders are brain disorders.

Another intuitive way of spelling out why physicalism seems to entail that all mental disorders are brain disorders is the following – if mental state A is identical with brain state α, then if mental state A is disordered/dysfunctional, then so is brain state α. After all, they are the same, so the same things are true of them. Note that this kind of argument presupposes the identity of mental and brain states. While most people assume that token brain states are identical with token mental states, type identity between mental states or processes and brain states or processes is widely thought to be much more doubtful.

Type identity may seem like too strong a relationship because of the possibility that one type of mental state may be realized by more than one type of brain state. Even so, one might be tempted by the following line of argument: given the dependence of the mental on the physical for its existence, every mental dysfunction depends on some corresponding underlying brain process for its realization. So, if the brain process is necessary for the mental dysfunction, and absent this brain process, we would not have a dysfunctional mental process; the brain process must also be dysfunctional.

But it is exactly this last claim, that the realizer inherits the properties of the realized property, that is controversial. Many philosophers and psychiatrists push back against the idea that any brain process which realizes a disordered mental process is *ipso facto* disordered. And indeed, Kendler himself points out that his claim that all mental disorders are biological is a very weak one. After all, according to physicalism, all mental processes are biological, so in that sense, there is nothing special about *disordered* mental processes. Like non-disordered mental processes, they are biological, in the sense that they require a biological organism to take place.[2]

This brings us to the key question: does the fact that, according to the   physicalist world-view, every disordered mental process requires a physical realizer – a brain state – to exist entail that this physical realizer itself is disordered or dysfunctional?

One could of course just claim that this is the case by metaphysical fiat. Whatever brain states underlie disordered mental states inherit the categorization as disordered. If the mind isn't doing what it should be doing, and the brain's function (among many others) is to produce mental states, then if it produces disordered mental states, it also is not doing what it should be doing. This solution has a certain elegance, but it is problematic; and many philosophers have dismissed it out of hand. I too believe that it is over-inclusive.

Why?

There are theoretical and practical objections, which are linked (cf. Jefferson 2021, 2020b, 2014). The primary theoretical objection points out that there may be different standards for what counts as pathological at the level of the brain and at the level of the mind. It is theoretically possible to say that the brain is functioning as it should, but things have gone wrong at the level of the mind. George Graham (2013b) presses this point. He claims that mental illness or disorder is not the same as brain disorder or disease: "They [mental disorders] are based in the brain, or *in* the brain as I like to put it, but not of the brain. They are not instances of a disordered brain" (Graham 2013b, 515). According to Graham, the brain can be doing exactly what it should be doing, while the mind is behaving in a dysfunctional way.

2.2.1 The hardware/software analogy

Assuming physicalism is true, what justifies a distinction between dysfunction at the level of the brain and dysfunction at the level of the mind? The term 'dysfunction' is certainly applicable at both levels. When blood flow in the brain is blocked in a stroke, this is an instance of dysfunction in the brain. What are our criteria for deciding when (if ever) dysfunction at the level of the mind also entails dysfunction in the underlying brain process? Most frequently, philosophers (and psychiatrists) draw an analogy to the hardware-software distinction in computers to make their case (Papineau 1994, Arpaly 2005, Kendler 2005, Cooper 2007, Graham 2013b).[3] They argue along the following lines:

when Bill performs a statistical analysis and gets the wrong results because there is a problem – a bug – in the software of his computer, that does not mean that there is a problem with the computer's hardware, even though all software requires hardware to run.

For the sake of precision and accuracy, it should be pointed out that the way the hardware/software relationship is portrayed in discussions in philosophy of psychiatry is overly simplistic. It is not the case that there are only two levels; the hardware level and the software level and identical software runs on different types of hardware. Rather, the software as programmed by the software engineers is compiled into software that the computer can read, and this compiled version is different between, for example, Macs and Windows PCs. So, in reality, different hardware *requires* different software. Nevertheless, we can hold on to the analogy as it is still true that, at the highest level, we have type identical software, even if it needs to be compiled into different instructions for different computers. And it is possible to have a problem in the code (software) without there being a technical defect in the hardware. So, the existence of a problem in the software does not entail the existence of a corresponding hardware problem.

Using analogical reasoning, philosophers have argued that the fact that there is a problem at the level of the mental does not entail that there is a problem at the level of the brain. Thus, the hardware/software distinction provides us with a model of how we can have dysfunction at the level of cognitive (mental) processes without having dysfunction at the level of physical (brain) processes. However, it turns out that the analogy falls down in a number of key respects: our criteria for establishing functionality at the hardware/software levels do not find a ready parallel in the case of the mind/brain. In order to see why this is the case, we need to dig a little bit deeper and see what the similarities and differences between the mind/brain and software/hardware are.

2.2.2 Multiple realizability

The hardware/software distinction is frequently employed by functionalist theories of the mind which clearly distinguish between properties at the mental and physical level. Functionalist theories individuate mental states by their functional role, the input and output conditions that they are associated with, rather than identifying them with the physical basis underlying these functional states.[4] To take the time-honoured example of pain, this is realized in different ways in octopuses and in humans, but as long as it is caused by damage to the body and leads to avoidance behaviour, it can still be classified as pain. Thus, functionalists can categorize things at the level of the mental independently of their classification at the level of the physical. Multiple realizability of mental states in different physical ways is often used to shore up this distinction. If pain can be realized in very different ways in an octopus and a human, then we cannot just make assumptions about the physical states of the octopus based on the fact that it is experiencing the same kind of mental state. Token mental and physical states are identical, but types are not.

Multiple realizability plays a slightly odd role in the debate about minds, brains, software and hardware. Functionalism is underwritten by multiple realizability and the analogy to the software/hardware distinction, too, is often supported by examples of multiple realization. One of the points of functionalism is that you can have something be mental state x irrespective of how it is physically realized. Similarly, the fact that one and the same software can run on different kinds of hardware (Macs and Windows PCs) is also an instance of the multiple realizability of that software. So, multiple realizability allows us to draw a distinction between the realizing property and the realized property. This might be the brain and the mind, or the hardware and the software. This is important in psychiatry, as it means that the level of the mental can be the right locus of scientific enquiry and theorizing, without scientists necessarily having to worry whether what is a unified phenomenon at the level of the mental is also a unified phenomenon at the level of the brain. This is sometimes called the autonomy of mental disorder – we can ascribe dysfunction and disorder at the level of the mind without knowing how this is realized at the level of the brain. But people who argue for the autonomy of mental disorders frequently make a further claim that mental disorders need not be brain disorders at all.[5]

It certainly seems that multiple realizability is sufficient to establish a hardware-software distinction. If one and the same program (type of mental state) runs on different kinds of hardware (brains) and is realized in very different ways on these, then it is clear that we should distinguish between the two, because identity of software properties does not carry over into identity of hardware properties. The alternative would be to say that anything that realizes a software problem is a hardware problem, and that certainly isn't what we say in the case of computers. But even though this sometimes gets muddled in the literature, the reason we do not say that every software problem is a hardware problem is not solely that software problems can be multiply realized; rather, we also appeal to other criteria.

2.2.3 Design specifications and difference makers

While philosophers make much of multiple realizability, computer engineers have further criteria for distinguishing between hardware and software problems in computers. They have factory specifications which state what the hardware is supposed to do and not to do. If it is not doing what it is specified to do, that counts as a hardware problem. Computers are artefacts, and as with other artefacts we have pre-existing definitions of what counts as functional and what doesn't. We design the hardware to be able to do certain things, and that determines its function. We don't have those functional specifications for the brain. This means that the main criterion for distinguishing between hardware and software malfunction, namely design specification or the intentions of the creator of an artefact, does not have a straightforward analogy for the brain/mind case.

A further difference between hardware and software problems philosophers and psychiatrists appeal to is that of difference makers. They point out that software and hardware problems arise in distinct ways and are fixed in distinct ways. If you have a hardware problem, you call the hardware engineer; if you have a software problem, the programmer needs to make some changes. This then shows that there are distinct problems at different levels, which have a different aetiology and are fixed (treated) in different ways (Papineau 1994, Kendler 2012). However, this supposed analogy does not hold, as we have seen in the previous chapter. Kendler (2012) points out that there are many difference makers at different levels in psychiatric illness, both when we look at the aetiology of disorders (risk factors) and at treatment options. For example, there are psychological, environmental, and biological risk factors for depression, and treatment can also target psychology, physiology or environment. Minds and brains are therefore disanalogous to software and hardware with respect to there being proprietary difference makers.

Incidentally, it should be noted that this is also a rather naive view of what is going on in the case of computers. There, too we have difference makers that cross the hardware/software distinction, as in the case where the Pentium bug (a hardware problem) was fixed with a software patch. Mind/brain and software/hardware are actually analogous in this respect: difference makers are not always what distinguishes a hardware problem from a software problem. This shows that 'how does it get fixed' is not a reliable criterion for distinguishing between hardware and software problems or mental dysfunction and brain dysfunction.

Looking at these similarities and differences between hardware/ software and brain/mind, it seems that a lot of the intuitive pull of employing the hardware–software distinction to show that mental dysfunction need not be brain dysfunction comes from the combination of multiple realizability and design specification. Multiple realizability gives us a rationale for saying that we can make generalizations at the level of the mental which do not have to carry down to the level of the brain. The difference in design process and intention gives us a way of specifying what the hardware is supposed to do and what the software is supposed to do in such a way that they can go wrong independently.

The hardware–software analogy is very compelling in providing a picture according to which things can go wrong independently of each other: if there is no common feature in the hardware of the PC and the Mac but the code is the same, and we can identify a problem in the code, it seems that there is a problem in the software, but not in the hardware. Accordingly, Cooper suggests that functionalism would lead to two different kinds of mental disorder: "Some would be caused by problems with the hardware of the brain. Others would be caused by problems in the software of the mind" (Cooper 2007, 110).

However, philosophers who employ the analogy to the hardware/ software distinction to show that mental disorders are not brain disorders ignore that we do not have different specifications for mind and brain in the way we have for computers. Furthermore, there are difference makers both at the level of the mind and at the level of the brain in mental disorders, so the analogy falls down there, too. This means that the computer analogy brings home something we found out via a different route in Chapter 2 – how hard it is to identify dysfunction at the level of the brain. Multiple realizability is the one factor left from the hardware/software analogy that plays a crucial role in denying that mental dysfunction entails brain dysfunction.

So, should we go all out physicalist and say that *whatever* realizes a dysfunctional mental process is *ipso facto* a disordered brain process? This would be a mistake. While the computer analogy cannot provide separate criteria of dysfunction for minds and brains in the way that we have for software and hardware, we also haven't established that we can just move from ascribing properties at the mental level to ascribing those same properties at the brain level.

For this, the possibility of multiple realizability matters. The conceptual point that functionalism allows us to distinguish between properties of minds and brains goes hand in hand with a practical objection against labelling each and every brain process underlying mental dysfunction as dysfunctional: we do not get any descriptive or explanatory mileage out of saying that a mental disorder is a brain disorder if we just make this a definitional issue. If the brain disorder label is that easy to come by, there is no requirement that there should be something systematic that is the same across the different brains that realize one and the same mental dysfunction.

In other words, if psychological dysfunction is very variably realized in different people's brains (or indeed, in the brain of one person over time), then calling the associated brain states or processes disordered is of no practical use whatsoever. What we want is a common brain process or structure that unites the brains of individuals suffering from a specific psychological dysfunction and distinguishes them from the brains of people who do not suffer from the psychological problem. This second part is important too. If we cannot distinguish the brains of people not suffering from mental dysfunction from those who do, then we do not have a basis for saying that we are dealing with brain dysfunction. (Though see Chapter 4 for some added complications.) We may think this is a non-problem, as surely there must be systematic differences to be found at the level of the brain when there are systematic mental differences. But brain science often struggles to show that brain differences we find at the group level between people with mental health conditions and the non-clinical population apply across the board. In other words, not every person who suffers from depression might have what is identified as a typical brain signature, and more worryingly, we may not be able to see any systematic differences between a person suffering from a condition and a healthy person. Some of the problems in identifying a brain signature are due to the fact that one and the same brain structure performs many functions (multifunctionality) and that one and the same function can be carried out by different regions (multiple realizability) (Pessoa 2019).

Unless we have an identifiable brain difference which is sufficient for brain dysfunction, we lack a scientifically useful feature that would justify speaking of brain disorders. We would instead be in the situation where the only reason we have for calling these brains disordered is a metaphysical commitment to physicalism together with the claim that the property of being disordered is inherited across levels of description. This is not to say that we cannot accommodate a certain amount of multiple realization – we may find that there are three 'kinds' of depression which are realized in three different ways. But dysfunction is a comparative term and therefore needs to be ascribed at the level of types of phenomena. In order to say that process x is dysfunctional, we need to have a systematic/repeating pattern that can be compared to a pattern of normal functioning. Too much variation undermines the identification of disordered types of brain processes. If we do not have any systematic brain signature, nothing would be gained by insisting that these disorders are brain disorders. Some authors claim that this is the case for depression (Borsboom, Cramer, and Kalis 2019).[6]

2.3 Interim summary

If we take paradigmatic neurodegenerative brain diseases as a model, mental disorders are not brain disorders, as discussed in the previous chapter. However, many mental disorders do respond to pharmacological treatment and involve brain difference, so if aetiology or treatment paths are considered deciding factors for classifying a condition as a brain disorder, some mental disorders will qualify. Criteria such as aetiology and treatment path do not give us a clearly delineated class of brain disorders, but rather, an overlap between mental disorders and brain disorders.

In this chapter, I have considered a different approach, which is to investigate whether certain views on the metaphysics of the mind–body relationship have implications for the mental dysfunction/brain dysfunction relationship, and consequently, for the mental disorder/brain disorder one. It turns out that contrary to popular belief, some forms of dualism are compatible with biological psychiatry and the claim that mental disorders are brain disorders. Physicalism, on the other hand, is compatible with a distinction between mental disorders and brain disorders, at least in principle. This has become obvious when we considered the claim that brain dysfunction is inherited from psychological dysfunction because of physicalism. If we take the view that every mental dysfunction is automatically a brain dysfunction (or that the existence of dysfunction in a psychological process entails dysfunction in the realizing process), we run the risk of losing any substantial notion of what it takes to be a brain disorder, especially if psychological dysfunction is realized in a plethora of different ways in different people and individuals across time. On this view, brain processes and states of a person suffering from a mental health condition would just be defined as pathological, without any guarantee that there will be anything substantial that brain research adds to describing and explaining the condition. I have also argued that while appeals to the hardware-software distinction and multiple realizability secure the idea that mental dysfunction need not entail brain dysfunction in the realizing brain states, it is unhelpful in telling us what to make of cases where mental dysfunction is indeed reliably realized by a specific brain process. One gets the impression that at least some philosophers hope that multiple realizability will guarantee that this question does not arise. What the discussion so far has also brought out is just how difficult the conceptual territory is. Metaphysical considerations regarding the mind-brain relationship do not give us a ready-made way of identifying which mental disorders are brain disorders unless we want to go for the theoretically dubious and scientifically useless claim that all mental disorders are brain disorders by definition. However, saying that brain disorders are just those ones where the brain is broken does not give us a workable notion of brain disorder either, because we need to establish *when* the brain is broken.

Another way of seeing this is by looking back at the point I made about criteria for dysfunctionality. In the case of the hardware-software distinction, we have the design purpose of the manufacturers or programmers. In the case of evolved organisms, some philosophers of biology and cognitive science respond that we have something similar in the case of the brain, which is evolved function (Fagerberg, 2022). Alternatively, we might think of dysfunction as mechanisms or traits not making the usual contribution to the system it is embedded in (Cummins 1975). Either of these notions of dysfunction requires a systematic difference at the level of the brain which holds across individuals. In the case of evolutionary accounts, we would need to establish the mechanisms of normal function and how this breaks down, and this requires systematic inter-individual patterns of function in order for us to say how the brain is supposed to work when performing a psychological process.[7] Similarly, in order to identify whether a process is not making its usual contribution to a psychological process, we need to know what the usual contribution is. So, dysfunction at the brain level requires identifiable patterns of function and dysfunction.

3 A middle way – being inclusive but not over-inclusive

The two definitions of brain dysfunction I have presented so far are either too narrow or over-inclusive. In Chapter 2, I argued that the notion of brain dysfunction and disorder based on paradigmatic cases is too restrictive, as it neglects the fact that for many mental and brain disorders physiological, psychological and environmental factors affect both the onset and the treatment of the condition. Furthermore, these accounts do not provide an account of brain dysfunction that goes beyond pointing to paradigm cases. We are given examples of what falls in the extension of 'brain disorder', but we are not told how to demarcate the extension. In this chapter, we have seen that going completely the other way and saying that all mental disorders are *ipso facto* brain disorders is also unsatisfactory, because considerations from multiple realizability leave open the in principle option that we will not find types of brain anomaly that are necessary for the occurrence of certain psychological dysfunctions. Mental dysfunction might be so multiply realized that we do not find an underlying brain pattern for a certain mental dysfunction. However, the preceding discussion also provides us with a criterion for saying when we are dealing with brain dysfunction. We should call those brain differences that reliably realize mental dysfunction brain dysfunctions. What does this mean?

Let's start with a definition:

It is sufficient for X to be a dysfunctional type of brain process if tokens of this type always realize a psychological dysfunction.

I specify this as a sufficiency condition because realization of psychological dysfunction is not the only kind of brain dysfunction. There can be antecedent brain dysfunctions that cause psychological dysfunction, such as for example brain tumours. There are also brain dysfunctions which cause perceptual or motor problems without necessary causing psychological dysfunction. These brain anomalies are all brain dysfunctions. *Our* question is how to extend the notion of brain dysfunction to those brain processes that realize the psychological dysfunctions we find in mental disorders.[8]

My inclusive view takes the threat from multiple realizability seriously and concedes that the possibility of widespread multiple realization shows that the existence of a certain type of mental dysfunction *does not entail* the existence of a corresponding brain dysfunction. However, the question to what extent mental disorders are multiply realized is an empirical question. Furthermore, as I have mentioned above and will expand on below, it is possible to accommodate a limited amount of multiple realization. Having more than one way of realizing a supervenient property is not a problem, as long as the realizing states or processes are not *too* variable. So this definition of brain dysfunction provides an answer to the unresolved question discussed above: what should we make of the cases where psychological dysfunction is realized in one way or a small number of tightly circumscribed ways?

My account provides a way of fleshing out an assumption that different accounts of brain disease share: a person is suffering from a brain disorder if it is correct to say that they are suffering from a harmful dysfunction (the disorder condition) and that there is something wrong with the *brain* (the brain dysfunction condition). On my account, we can establish harmful dysfunction on the psychological level and label abnormal brain processes that instantiate these psychological dysfunctions as dysfunctional. In these cases, both the epistemology and the metaphysics go from the mind to the brain. As Schramme (2013) puts it, mental disorders are autonomous, they do not rely on dysfunction in the brain for their status as disorders. But my claim is that this autonomy is compatible with cases of brain dysfunction which are pathological precisely because these types of brain processes instantiate a type of psychological dysfunction. We find out which brain differences are dysfunctions by finding out what psychological processes they realize, and they are brain dysfunctions because they realize psychological dysfunction. As mentioned above, there are other forms of brain pathology. For example, a brain tumour that only affected the motor system would still be pathological. When tumours do lead to psychological dysfunction, they causally precede it. But being a type of brain process that realizes a type of psychological dysfunction is one way of being a brain dysfunction. And the mental disorder which involves this brain dysfunction is also a brain disorder.

We can think of this as a response to the hardware/software objection to identifying mental disorders with brain disorders. I have argued that the analogy between minds and computers has been overstated. But it does make conceptual space for mental disorders which are not brain disorders in those cases where there are no specific brain differences that set people suffering from the disorder apart from people in the non-clinical population. However, it *also* makes conceptual space for mental disorders which are brain disorders. It is possible that scientists do find these systematic brain differences. Assume, for the sake of argument, that we find differences in the dopamine system in addiction that underlie the cravings for the drug that we are familiar with on the psychological level and that we have characterized as dysfunctional psychological processes. There is promising research in this area (Holton and Berridge 2013).[9] Let us further assume that these differences in brain function are sufficient for the cravings, that we will not find this kind of brain difference without cravings. This means that this pattern of brain function realizes cravings. In other words, it fulfils the condition of being sufficient for mental dysfunction and realizing that dysfunction specified above. This would then be a case where a mental dysfunction is also a brain dysfunction. On the assumption that disorders involving brain dysfunction are brain disorders, we should further conclude that we are dealing with a brain disorder.

Note that it is in principle possible (and likely to be the case) that one and the same psychological dysfunction can be realized by more than one brain anomaly. Consider a scenario where there are three different types of brain anomalies which realize cravings. I see no in principle reason to deny that all three types of brain anomaly count as dysfunctional. This is not a problem for the account as long as (a) realizers don't proliferate (if they did, explanatory and descriptive usefulness would be lost) and (b) we do not get the brain anomaly without the psychological one, i.e., the specific pattern of brain function is sufficient for the psychological dysfunction. But as the example has shown, the existence of brain anomaly x need not be a necessary condition for psychological dysfunction χ. It could be that χ is realized by a different brain anomaly y. For example, some studies suggest that depression involves different types of activation patterns in different patient populations and that these different activation patterns are predictive of what kind of treatment will work for patients (Roiser, Elliott, and Sahakian 2012, Nord et al. 2019). This provides early stage evidence that there may be different but identifiable types of brain dysfunction that realize dysfunctional mental processes we find in depression. It should however be noted that what this study identified as a biomarker for depression was a difference in activation patterns in the brain in depressed patients which was not tied to a dysfunctional psychological process as such, but measured different patterns of activation in cognitive tasks, such as working memory tasks.

There are a number of objections to the account I propose, which I will consider as a way of clarifying and strengthening it in the following chapters. But before doing so, I will highlight a strength of my account. It allows us to make sense of the claim by the NIMH (The US National Institute of Mental Health) that mental disorders are brain disorders. Thomas Insel, former head of the NIMH has argued that mental disorders are brain disorders and urged a departure from DSM style symptom-based classification. Instead of using the DSM, the NIMH proposes that we should focus on areas of functioning. Two things will become clear in looking at the NIMH's Research Domain Criteria (abbreviated RDoC) and comparing it with my account: (1) my definition of brain dysfunction can make good sense of an existing research model in the neurosciences and provide it with theoretical grounding. However, (2) the notion of disorder entailed, based on dysfunction of psychological and brain processes, departs quite radically from classic nosological categories (for example 'depression', 'schizophrenia', etc.).

3.1 Mental disorders as brain disorders – the RDoC

Proponents of the RDoC framework designed it to guide mental health research and its authors have prominently claimed that mental disorders are indeed brain disorders. What do they mean by that? Bolton (2013) points out that this is not a reductionist project,[10] where by reductionism he means that *all* explanatory (or causal) power is located at the level of the brain. Rather, the RDoC explicitly allows for a multi-causal nexus of different factors affecting both the onset and the treatment of mental health conditions. The programme was (and is) driven by dissatisfaction with existing, syndrome-based method of mental health categorization. Syndrome-based categorization such as that used in the DSM diagnoses a mental health condition on the basis of a normally disjunctive set of symptoms. The criteria for Major Depressive Disorder (MDD) include: depressed mood, lack of interest and pleasure in everyday activities, weight loss or weight gain, inability to sleep/sleeping a lot, psycho-motor agitation or retardation, fatigue, feelings of worthlessness and guilt, diminished ability to concentrate, recurrent thoughts of death or suicidal ideation. A person will meet the diagnostic criteria for depres-sion if five or more symptoms are present, with depressed mood or lack of interest and pleasure having to be one of the symptoms (APA 2013, 160–161). This method of diagnosis and categorization can group a very heterogenous set of people as suffering from the same condition. Some of these people may exhibit significant differences in symptoms, even if there is a recognizable pattern. (There are 256 symptom combinations. Given that depressed mood or lack of interest or pleasure need to be present, this leaves 227 ways of meeting the diagnostic criteria. The fact that some symptoms can be realized in more than one way – weight loss *or* weight gain – adds even further variability. As a matter of fact, not all of these combinations tend to occur and there are recognizable symptom clusters, but there is still considerable variation (Zimmerman et al. 2015, 30).[11]) A further worry about current diagnostic categories is that individuals frequently also suffer from comorbidity, where they are diagnosed with more than one syndrome-based disorder.

> [P]atients who meet criteria for one mental disorder often tend to meet criteria for other mental disorders – a phenomenon known as **comorbidity.** This has led researchers to question whether too much emphasis has been placed on studying specific disorders in isolation from other disorders. It has also led to concerns that com-mon dimensions underlying mental disorders are not being prop-erly reflected in mental health research.
>
> (NIMH)

Researchers and clinicians worry that rather than comorbidity genu-inely being the result of different problems, diagnostic categories don't match the underlying problems, such that there is double counting of one and the same psychological dysfunction which leads to two different diagnoses.

Instead of syndrome-based diagnoses, the RDoC operates with six domains of human functioning as the focus of inquiry. These are: negative valence, positive valence, cognitive systems, systems for social processes, arousal regulatory systems, sensorimotor systems. These domains then break up into lots of sub-domains (for example, for cognitive systems, we have, among others, declarative memory, working memory, cognitive control). The framework then looks at these domains of functioning using different units of analysis (neural) circuits, behaviour, physiology and self-report, utilizing information at many different levels.

One underlying stated ambition of the RDoC, which has generated much controversy, is to find out what is going wrong in the brain when people suffer from mental disorders. Proponents of the RDoC claim that it is not terribly surprising that our disorder categorizations aren't much good, because they do not look at the underlying 'pathophysiological mechanisms' (Insel et al. 2010, 748). Importantly for the issues discussed above, the RDoC also rejects the lesion-based account we find in Szasz and instead favours a broader notion of brain dysfunction: "In contrast to neurological disorders with identifiable lesions, mental disorders can be addressed as disorders of brain circuits" (Insel et al. 2010, 749). This shows that a notion of brain dysfunction as 'brain difference that realizes psychological dysfunction' is already implicitly at work in biomedical research. This matters because many psychologists, psychiatrists and philosophers write as though a narrow Szasz-style, lesion-based understanding of brain pathology and dysfunction were the only theoretical option.

Another important thing to bear in mind is that, rhetoric notwithstanding, this is a research programme. It hopes to find systematic brain differences for dysfunctional processes at the psychological level, but that is a mission statement, not an existing result.[12] Much of the resistance to RDoC results not so much from the scientific goals, but from a rhetoric and swagger that suggest that these goals have already been met. I agree with the RDoC in that I believe it *could* turn out that all mental disorders are brain disorders. It is conceivable that we will find brain processes that underlie the mental dysfunctions in all mental disorders. But in order to establish whether this is the case, we need to show that dysfunctional psychological processes are realized by types of brain processes which can be distinguished from normal functioning processes. There are some areas where progress on this kind of project is being made – thus, for example, finding realizers for overactive fear responses in anxiety and panic disorders would establish brain dysfunction in these conditions, and there is progress in finding such underlying brain dysfunction that realizes these fear responses (de Carvalho, Rozenthal, and Nardi 2010).

4 Conclusion

I have proposed an inclusive account of brain dysfunction which allows us to say that mental disorders involve brain dysfunction (and are therefore brain disorders) provided certain conditions are met: there is an anomaly in brain structure or function that either causes or realizes the psychological dysfunction that leads us to posit a mental illness. I have also argued that, rather than being a purely theoretical exercise, this notion of brain dysfunction could underwrite the understanding of brain disorder found in a prominent research project, the RDoC. While I do not accept the claim that physicalism entails that all mental disorders are necessarily brain disorders, my account is more closely aligned with the over-inclusive view than with the narrow view. I accept the possibility that all mental disorders are brain disorders, but in order to show that this is the case for any given condition, we need to be able to show that, and how, specific brain differences realize psychological dysfunction.

One other thing this chapter achieves is to show why the chasm between proponents of the narrow view and those who lean towards the view that physicalism implies that all mental disorders are brain disorders is so wide and deep. When a proponent of the over-inclusive view says that mental disorders are brain disorders, they aren't actually saying anything that is empirically testable or would make a difference to our understanding of the condition. They are simply stating what they believe to be a straightforward equivalence which follows from a materialist world-view. This is the reason why I insist on something more demanding: stable realizing processes. However, there are a number of objections which need to be answered before we can accept my account.

I have argued that we are dealing with a brain dysfunction if a certain brain anomaly invariably realizes a certain psychological dysfunction. But what should we say if there were cases where one and the same psychological process counts as dysfunctional in one context but not in another? This problem is discussed under the heading of externalism in the philosophy of psychiatry. For example, it has been argued that the brain changes and psychological cravings we find in addiction can also be found in processes that we take to be non-pathological, for example when newly in love (Lewis 2017).

A further possible objection is that even if the project of finding brain dysfunctions for specific psychological processes is successful, brain dysfunction will be categorized at the symptom level by picking out a disordered psychological process, whereas mental disorders still get categorized at the symptom cluster level. Even if a cluster involves some identifiable brain dysfunction, this may not be the case across symptoms. So saying that the condition is a brain disorder would wrongly suggest some kind of unity that does not in fact exist. I will discuss these and other problems in the following chapter.

Notes

1 The kind of dualism most psychiatrists object to as incompatible with biological psychiatry is substance dualism. While substance dualism is indeed a niche position these days, Rachel Cooper (2007) argues that even on a Cartesian, substance dualist account, brain processes are thought to influence the mind. Thus, Descartes was aware that getting drunk will affect one's mood via one's physiology (Cooper 2007, 107). I myself doubt that Descartes's own dualism, which sees reasoning and thinking as a purely mental process independent of the body – albeit relying on sensory input from the body – is compatible with biological psychiatry and modern neuroscience.

2 Cf. Arpaly (2005) for a similar argument.

3 Not everyone appeals to the hardware/software distinction. Schramme (2013) appeals to multiple realization of mental states to argue against type identity of mental and brain states and against the unquestioning inference that mental disorders are automatically brain disorders.

4 As Cooper (2007) points out, functionalism is not necessarily a materialist/physicalist theory. While most functionalists are also physicalists, they need not be. In principle, the soul could realize functional states, though it is not obvious how we'd draw a distinction between the soul and the mental states it realizes.

5 Some even go so far as to say that mental dysfunction and brain dysfunction are dichotomous: a condition can be either a mental disorder or a brain disorder, but not both (Graham 2013b). But this argument would only appear to go through if it were the case that the hardware/software distinction and the brain/mind distinction rely exclusively on multiple realizability and dysfunctional mental processes are indeed multiply realized in humans.

6 I would like to thank Kengo Miyazono and Harriet Fagerberg for pressing me on whether multiple realizability really matters.

7 Harriet Fagerberg (2022) disagrees. She argues that both mental functions and brain functions are evolved functions and that mental dysfunction can be multiply realized by different patterns of brain dysfunction. I remain unconvinced. If both functional mental processes and dysfunctional ones can have a wide variety of realizing patterns, this precludes establishing a pattern of normal functioning. This theoretical disagreement may not matter much in practice – if we do find systematic patterns for function and dysfunction, our accounts will coincide.

8 The account put forward here is a development of the position I first introduce in (Jefferson 2020b). I also give an overview of my position for a more general audience in Jefferson (2021).

9 Though see Marc Lewis (2017) and the discussion in the next chapter for a view that brain processes in addiction are not qualitatively different from those found in other reward learning processes.

10 As I will argue in the next chapter, this is a rather non-standard use of the term 'reduction' in philosophy of science, but it's used more frequently in the psychiatry and clinical psychology literature.

11 The cited study by Zimmerman et al., which looks at the different symptom variations found, draws on the DSMIV, but there are still nine items in the diagnostic criteria for Major Depressive Disorder in the DSM5, which have remained largely the same.

12 Cf. Jurjako and Malatesti (2020) on the RDoC's brain disorder claim being a methodological move along the lines of Carnapian explication.

4 Objections and clarifications

1 Introduction

There are important objections that need to be addressed in order to defend the inclusive view of brain disorders; doing this will also clarify it further. The first is the reductionism objection. A common objection to the claim that (some) mental disorders are brain disorders is that this claim is committed to an unfeasible form of reductionism. This objection was recently raised again in a prominent paper by Denny Borsboom and colleagues, who object to the claim that mental disorders are brain disorders, in particular as championed by the RDoC project. I show that objections to reductionism frequently conflate different kinds of reduction, and that while my account is committed to one of them, explanatory reduction, it is not committed to the more problematic one, which I will give the rather clunky name 'single brain cause aetiology reduction'. Furthermore, arguments to the effect that reduction of mental dysfunction to brain dysfunction is *in principle impossible* are unconvincing.

A further objection against biological psychiatry stems from the claim that psychiatry is externalist in important ways, but biological psychiatry and brain disorders presuppose internalism. From this, it supposedly follows that biological psychiatry and the hypothesis that mental disorders are brain disorders are doomed because both presuppose an internalist understanding of disorder which does not apply in the case of mental disorders. Philosophers have indeed convincingly argued that the decision whether a certain condition or symptom counts as pathological is partially externalist in the following sense: contextual and historical factors determine whether, for example, low mood counts as dysfunctional or not. If this is true, it raises the questions whether (a) something counting as a brain dysfunction is also context dependent and (b) whether this is a problem for my view.

DOI: 10.4324/9780367822088-4

In this chapter, I will outline the reductionism objection and show that the form of reductionism my account is committed to is unproblematic. I will then address the externalism objection. I concede that the interaction between the agent and their environment plays an important role in deciding which conditions are pathological. However, this is also the case for somatic disorders, so all disorders are somewhat externalist. Furthermore, the case for the externalism of mental disorders has been overstated; mental disorders still presuppose some level of internal dysfunction, even if this is defined in part by appeal to appropriate reactions to external stimuli.

2 The reductionism objection

Worries about reductionism feature prominently in objections to the claim that mental disorders are brain disorders, though they take different forms. As different authors have different targets in mind when they worry about reductionism, it is worth looking closely at the specific objections that are raised. Recently, Borsboom and colleagues (2019) have objected to the RDoC's goal of identifying mental disorders with brain disorders on the grounds that it is committed to an unfeasibly reductionist agenda. They claim that an approach which defines mental disorders as brain disorders necessarily and essentially aims at reduction. It follows that *if* you cannot reduce mental processes to brain processes, mental disorders cannot be brain disorders.

One might think that all this amounts to is that Borsboom make the rather sensible assertion that unless we have evidence of reducibility of mental dysfunction to brain dysfunction, it's an open empirical question whether mental disorders like depression are brain disorders. In that case, claiming that they are would be premature. This would be a sensible, cautious line of argument that I would agree with. It is also one point they make in their paper. However, the authors pursue a more ambitious project, as is already indicated in the paper's title: "Brain disorders? Not really: why network structures *block* reductionism in psychopathology reseach" (emphasis added). They assert that mental disorders are not brain disorders, because they are not reducible, due to their network structure. (The idea being that mental disorders are constituted by symptom clusters, which act as a mutually reinforcing network.)[1] Why are Borsboom and colleagues so confident about the non-reducibility of mental disorders? Let us look at what they say:

> Many believe that symptoms, signs, and other problems associated with mental disorders – for example, depressed mood, psychomotor

agitation – are caused by "genes for mental disorders," neurobio-logical mechanisms, deficient brain circuits, and other biological factors. This firm belief in explanatory reductionism – that is, the belief that mental disorders can be explained ultimately in terms of specific dysfunctional neurobiological conditions – is partly be-cause the study of mental disorders traditionally belonged to the medical discipline. (…) Currently, there is no compelling evidence for the viability of reducing mental disorders to unique biological abnormalities, both in terms of enhanced etiological understanding and of improving the effectiveness of interventions.

(Borsboom et al. 2019, 1–2)

This quote throws up three questions:

1 What do Borsboom et al. mean by reduction? We have already seen in the previous chapter that this term has a multitude of uses in the literature.
2 Do accounts which take mental disorders to be brain disorders aim at reduction? Clearly, the answer to this question will depend on the answer to the first question.
3 Is it impossible to reduce dysfunctional mental processes to dys-functional brain processes and are we in a position to know this?

2.1 What kind of reductionism?

As we have seen, there are different forms of reductionism at play in discussions in the philosophy of science and mind. Ontological reductionism, the claim that mental processes are at base brain processes does not seem to be what Borsboom et al. have in mind. Rather, they explicitly target explanatory (epistemological) reductionism. To add to the terminological abundance, this form of reduction is also called scien-tific reduction, because phenomena which are described in one scientific theory are reduced to the entities which are described and theorized in a lower level science, with physics being the lowest level science.

One classic example of reduction is the identification of temperature with kinetic energy. At its most ambitious, reductionism aims to reduce everything to physics, as the fundamental science. Thus, for example, Bolton and Gillett understand physicalism and reductionism to go hand in hand, and characterize the reductionist project as follows: "all causa-tion and all causal laws are physical, or another way of putting this: physics explains everything" (Bolton and Gillett 2019, 59). Bolton and Gillett's understanding of reductionism is somewhat non-standard in that they take the reductionist project to be an eliminativist one, which characterizes the (to be) reduced level as unreal. However, normally scientific or explanatory reduction is conservative, it takes the reduced level and its phenomena to be real, even if they can be translated into the language of the underlying science. While classic explanatory reductionism is indeed reduction to physics, this is not the kind of reductionism at play in debates about mental disorders, brain disorders and reduction. In this context, the reducing level is that of brain processes, biology and physiology.[2] Psychological phenomena are to be reduced to neuroscientific ones.

On my account, successful explanatory reduction is indeed a precondition for calling a mental dysfunction a brain dysfunction, because I defined brain dysfunctions as those brain processes that instantiate the corresponding mental dysfunction. If there are no systematic brain anomalies that instantiate mental dysfunction, there is no case for brain dysfunction, because brain dysfunction is a property of types of brain states. The same line of reasoning holds for the RDoC, which talks of mental disorders as disorders of brain circuits. So it is correct that the brain disorder account entails explanatory reductionism. However, a closer look at Borsboom et al. shows that the reductionist agenda they ascribe to projects like the RDoC is somewhat more ambitious.

How so? There is a recurring use of the word 'reduction' in psychiatry and the philosophy of psychiatry that understands reductive explanations in psychiatry as those which posit some kind of *preceding* brain defect which is the (single) cause of mental dysfunction. To see this, let us have a quick look back at the quote I first introduced. Borsboom et al. state that "currently, there is no compelling evidence for the viability of reducing mental disorders to unique biological abnormalities, both in terms of enhanced etiological understanding and of improving the effectiveness of interventions" (Borsboom, Cramer, and Kalis 2019, 1–2).

The focus on aetiology shows that we are again dealing with the idea we can find a preceding brain cause. Borsboom et al. identify the goal of explanatory reduction as the aim "to identify a common pathogenic pathway at the level of the brain that causally explains symptom patterns" (3). What this quote suggests is that reduction as required by the brain disorder model gives us both one common underlying cause (as in the syphilis model we have already encountered) and that this cause is located in the brain. For the record, it is important to note that Borsboom and colleagues object to two separate claims that they see the brain disorder account as committed to. They disagree with the latent variable approach to mental disorder, where the assumption is that there is one common underlying cause to illness. Instead, they conceive mental disorders as symptoms of mutually reinforcing clusters. Additionally, they see the brain disorder account as committed to that latent variable being a *brain dysfunction*. In essence, they see the brain disorder account to be committed to the idea that there is a single brain cause for mental disorder, a form of reductionism we can call 'single cause aetiology reduction'. (In Radden's terminology of medical imaginaries as models of psychiatric disorders, we can call this the neurosyphilis model, where there is one underlying causal pathway in the body.)

This way of understanding reduction as the process of finding *prior* causes for mental disorders in the brain can also be found in Mitchell (2012) and Bolton (2013). However, unlike Borsboom et al., Bolton does not interpret the RDoC's claim that mental disorders are brain disorders to be reductionist in this sense.

> While this proposal [that mental disorders are brain disorders] is not new, what is striking is that these two recent formulations are plainly not reductionist. By this, I mean that they do not suppose that neural dysfunctions are the only causes of mental disorders, but rather recognize developments in mental health sciences showing that causes or risks of mental disorders may operate at many levels, including the genetic and the neural, the individual, the family environment, and the social context.
>
> (Bolton 2013, 24)

In talking about reductionism in psychiatry there is often some slippage. Kendler (2005) correctly states that many reductionist projects see the reducing level as privileged, some even dispute the reality of the (to be) reduced psychological phenomena and processes. It is then a short step to the characterization of reductionism as one where only brain aetiologies count.

In talking about reductionism in psychiatry, one needs to acknowledge an important difference between causes that can be *described* at the level of the brain and causes that are, as it were, non-psychological. A bacterial infection is non-psychological, even though it will lead to brain changes which realize psychological changes. However, post-traumatic stress disorder (PTSD) will also involve brain changes in response to a traumatic event that realize psychological changes. The experiences that constitute the cause for PTSD as well as the psychological processes that constitute the dysfunction in PTSD are all realized in the brain. But this does not mean that the condition was not caused by a traumatic psychological event, nor that we can usefully exchange the psychological explanation with a neurological one, *even though the psychological causes obviously required a neurological realization.* At every step of the way, there will be brain processes realizing the psychological processes. PTSD is a quintessentially psychologically caused condition because it is, by definition, a response to traumatic life events. But it is also a disorder where the symptoms of the condition are associated with well-explored changes in brain chemistry and functional activation patterns in the brain. Thus, hyper-arousal is associated with specific differences in amygdala function, and there are a number of changes in the production and uptake of hormones such as cortisol (cf. Yehuda et al. 2015). It is this reduction of dysfunctional psychological processes to differences in brain function that explanatory reductionism strives for. However, Borsboom et al. see the RDoC specifically, and the brain disorder view more generally, as committed to a view which conflates two forms of reductionism – reductionism as cross-level identification and reductionism as identifying causal aetiology in the brain. This conflation is unfortunate but not uncommon, as we have already seen in the context of a Szaszian, strong reading of 'brain disorder'. But objections arising from the reading of reductionism as single brain cause aetiology reductionism do not apply to my account, because finding a preceding brain cause is not a necessary feature of brain dysfunction.

Contrary to what Borsboom and colleagues suggest, these objections also do not apply to accounts like the RDoC, which is commonly accused of being overly reductionist in its aims. The RDoC is explicitly not committed to a single cause aetiology model. It is obviously possible that for some conditions there will be preceding brain causes as well as reducibility. But having a clearly physiological pathology that exists prior to any psychological dysfunction is just one way of being a brain disorder, on my account. If the biological processes underlying dysfunctional psychological processes in PTSD can be elucidated, then we can speak of this as a disorder involving brain dysfunction, and therefore a brain disorder. There is more than one way of being a brain disorder, and more than one way of identifying pathology in the brain.

Admittedly, associations with the syphilis model of brain disorders are strong, and this means that people often associate single cause aetiology models with the term 'brain disorder'. But in as far as we understand brain disorders as conditions involving dysfunction at the level of the brain, there is no reason to do this. The very least critics of brain disorder views should do is to take the explicit commitments of the positions they are attacking seriously. In the case of Borsboom et al., this would have meant acknowledging that approaches like the RDoC are not committed to a single brain cause aetiology. It is then still open to critics to say that their own use of the term 'brain disorder' is more in keeping with common use. It is however doubtful that there is one such shared, common understanding of the term, and that in itself is a big part of the problem.

2.2 Objections to explanatory reduction

I have shown that, in one respect, the characterization of the mental disorders as brain disorders view provided by Borsboom et al. misses the target. But that of course leaves open the option that the goal of explanatory reduction may also be impossible. I explicitly allow for the possibility that we may not find systematic brain differences that realize mental dysfunction and that reduction may therefore be impossible. Whether all mental disorders are brain disorders is an empirical question. However, Borsboom and colleagues argue for an in-principle impossibility. Their first argument is that their understanding of disorders as mutually reinforcing symptom clusters makes it impossible for mental disorders to be brain disorders. The second is that our classification of certain mental states as disordered relies on their content, and that mental content is unlikely to be reducible. What should we make of these arguments?

2.2.1 Symptom clusters and reduction

Borsboom et al. rightly claim that current mental disorders are not well explained as stemming from one unified underlying brain cause (the neurosyphilis model). Rather, they conceptualize disorders as a set of mutually reinforcing symptom clusters. They concede that it is in principle conceivable that one might find an underlying realizer for each of the different symptoms, rather than one unified common cause that can be identified at the level of the brain. They then go on to claim that it is unlikely to be the case that we can do this across all symptoms. According to Borsboom et al., some symptoms will be too multiply realized to be reducible. In particular, they pick out the content of mental symptoms as something that will not be reducible, and then go on to argue that, particularly in the case of delusions, we often appeal to content to classify a certain belief as pathological.

For this to constitute a good objection to the brain disorder view, it needs to be the case that complete reduction of a condition is needed in order to call it a brain disorder. If we establish that a condition involves dysfunctional brain processes as part of the package, why should that not be sufficient for calling it a brain disorder? The main reason I can see against this approach is that people will jump to something like the single cause picture when they hear that x is a brain disorder. But we have already established that this is not a good model for most mental health conditions. There is no in principle reason why a psychiatric disorder shouldn't be a brain disorder because it involves brain dysfunction. Alternatively, we might conclude that the real problem is that current classification lumps too disparate a set of phenomena together as one condition and should be overhauled. This certainly is the direction in which the RDoC is moving when it aims to identify specific (mental or brain) dysfunctions rather than retaining the classic disorders. It therefore looks as though Borsboom et al. are attacking the project for something it is not aiming to do, which is to give a reductionist explanation of mental disorders while retaining current classifications. The very impetus to classify by areas of functioning rather than by mental disorders stems from the perception that symptom clusters are not the way forward in a reductionist project.

2.2.2 Multiple realizability – again

I now want to turn to Borsboom et al.'s objections to reduction on the basis of multiple realizability. Like many others in the debate, they make multiple realizability central to their argument, claiming that multiple realization makes reduction impossible.

We have already seen in the discussion in the previous chapter that a certain amount of multiple realization is compatible with reduction.[3] We can have more than one realization base. Tuomas Pernu (2019) makes this point specifically for criticism of the RDoC. Lack of fit with current classifications should not be seen as an objection to the RDoC's reductionist project. If it turns out that one kind of mental disorder identified by current classificatory means such as the DSM5 is realized in different ways in the brain, one possible conclusion is that we are dealing with more than one dysfunction rather than giving up on the reduction in psychiatry.

But maybe Borsboom and colleagues are making a stronger claim, namely that no systematic brain differences that hold across groups of individuals can be found. They rightly point out that the content of beliefs or desires is often relevant when saying that certain beliefs are symptoms of a disorder. So, for example, delusions are particularly bizarre or unlikely beliefs. They then also say that a specific belief content is more likely than not multiply realized. For example, it will be hard to find a single type of realizer for the belief that one's husband has been replaced by an imposter. I agree with the claim that we are unlikely to be able to reduce individual beliefs. However, reduction of the content of individual mental states is not the kind of reduction at stake. Why not? It is true that content plays a role in identifying a belief as a delusion, though it is far from the only criterion, so in assessing whether certain beliefs are delusions, we look at the content. However, a bizarre false belief is not in and of itself a clinical symptom. For a belief to count as pathological or a manifestation of pathology, it needs to be the case that this belief is largely resistant to counter-evidence and is not easily explained by the evidence available to the person. People who have bizarre beliefs because they inhabit a particularly esoteric epistemic bubble are not considered to be exhibiting pathological delusions, though their beliefs may be both bizarre and undesirable. When it comes to ascribing psychological dysfunction, we look at processes of belief formation and maintenance (Bortolotti and Miyazono 2015). And it is these kinds of patterns of perception, belief formation and belief maintenance that are classified as dysfunctional at the psychological level and the level of the brain. While the content of certain beliefs is an important indicator that something unusual may be going on in the way beliefs are formed, specific contents are neither necessary nor sufficient for calling a certain belief delusional. What a focus on how certain mental phenomena are characterized as pathological does show is that the level of description which tracks normative criteria such as rationality is not eliminable. But it was already conceded in the previous chapter's discussion that the psychological will continue to play a key role, as dysfunctionality criteria are inherited from that level.[4]

To conclude – the reduction objection stems in part from the terminological conflation of different ideas: the idea that reduction shows a single cause brain aetiology and the idea that reduction involves cross-level identification (explanatory reduction). The former is not required by the account and should in any case be kept conceptually separate. The latter is indeed implied and cannot simply be shown to be impossible by gesturing to multiple realizability. Furthermore, the fact that we use belief content in assessing whether certain beliefs are likely to be delusional in nature does not show that we need to be able to reduce individual beliefs. What it does show is that the psychological level, which employs normative notions of 'normal' or appropriate belief formation processes or emotional reactions does not become redundant.

3 The externalism worry

Will Davies has raised a further worry concerning biological psychiatry and brain disorder accounts of mental illness; he argues that the relationship to the external world is of key importance in classifying a condition as a mental disorder in a way that isn't the case for somatic disorders. So, whether a mental process or phenomenon is pathological depends not just on the internal states of the person affected, but on the interaction between internal states and environment. For example, Horwitz and Wakefield have argued that whether or not low mood should count as pathological depends on whether it is an expectable and proportionate response to adverse life events (Horwitz and Wakefield 2007).

Externalism is used as an objection against bio-medical psychiatry, with the brain disorder view of mental disorders considered one tenet of biomedical psychiatry. As the term 'bio-medical psychiatry' is as badly defined as the notion of a brain disorder, I will just go straight to the question whether externalist considerations show us that mental disorders cannot be brain disorders.

The externalist objection against the brain disorder view holds that mental disorders are fundamentally different from somatic disorders in their dependence on environmental factors, and therefore cannot be brain disorders. In answering this objection, I argue that the difference between psychiatric and somatic disorders has been overstated, as has been the degree to which psychiatric conditions are externalist. First, there are externalist criteria for the individuation of all disorders, be they psychiatric or somatic. This means that psychiatric disorders are not uniquely special in being externalist, and there is thus no fundamental difference between somatic disorders and psychiatric ones in this respect. However, the level of externalism described by Davies (2016) in his argument for externalist psychiatry seems to go beyond what we see in other forms of disorder. My second response therefore targets Davies' characterization of the level of externalism we find in mental illness. His claims are not borne out by the way psychiatry classifies mental disorders, there are still relevant internal differences between disordered states and qualitatively similar non-clinical ones.

3.1 Externalism in psychiatry

The term 'externalism' is used in so many different ways in the philosophy of mind and, more recently, psychiatry (Davies 2016, Glackin 2017, Roberts, Krueger, and Glackin 2019), that when a person says that they hold an externalist view of the status or constitution of mental disorders, this does not pinpoint their commitments very precisely. At its most general, externalism in psychiatry (and, indeed, in medicine more broadly) holds that factors outside the individual matter to (a) the classification of a condition as a certain disorder, for example, PTSD, or (b) deciding whether a certain mental phenomenon counts as disordered rather than healthy. In the first case, external factors matter to what type of condition we are dealing with, in the second to its status as pathological. It is the second question that is of primary importance for me, but it is useful to be aware that there are different forms of externalism, which pinpoint different ways in which the relationship between organism and external world plays a role in psychiatry. There are many ways in which the external world plays a role in the classification and constitution of mental disorders. In a recent paper, Tom Roberts, Shane Glackin and Joel Kruger (2019) enumerate six (!) different kinds of externalism that are relevant in psychiatry. Rather than running through all of these, I will give a general characterization and then focus on some relevant types of externalism.

Some externalist claims can be fairly uncontroversial or even trivial, for example, causal externalism points to the fact that certain environmental factors may be responsible for the onset of a mental disorder. We will ignore these kinds of factors because it's well established that environmental factors play a key causal role in both somatic and psychiatric conditions. Samei Huda (2019, 224 and 227) cites evidence that loneliness is associated with a higher risk of cardiovascular disease and stroke, and that there is a link between childhood adversity and inflammatory markers. On the uncontroversial assumption that environmental factors contribute to ill health as well as internal ones, causal externalism features in both somatic and psychiatric disorders.

The kind of externalism I am interested in here is one where the status of a phenomenon as pathological depends on the interaction between the individual and their environment. Davies (2016) draws attention to the fact that judgements of disorderedness involve an *appropriateness criterion*; they characterize a psychological pattern as disordered on the basis that it is a disproportionate response to environmental stimuli. "Depression crucially involves states that are unwarranted by or disproportionate to events in the subject's life. Aristotle thus characterized 'melancholia' as a sadness that is 'cold beyond due measure', producing a 'groundless despondency'" (Davies 2016, 293).

It is important to distinguish these kinds of cases where pathology depends on whether the psychological phenomena are appropriate given external events from cases where the cause of the disorder is part of its classification. A diagnosis of PTSD requires that there have been a precipitating traumatic event (APA 2013, 271). But the fact that it is a reaction to a traumatic event is not in itself what makes the condition disordered. Similar psychological phenomena without the precipitating cause would be just as pathological. We have similar ways of classifying somatic disorders by their causes. For example, Shane Glackin (2017) points out that pneumonia is often classified by its aetiology (viral, bacterial, fungal) or even by the circumstances in which it was acquired (community acquired, hospital acquired, ventilator associated). Both somatic medicine and psychiatry sometimes use aetiology to classify conditions, without this being the way we decide whether a condition is pathological or not in the first place. In the following, the focus will be on cases where the judgement of disorderedness itself depends on the organism-environment interaction.

Davies (2016) has argued that externalism sets psychiatric disorders (mental health conditions) apart from somatic disorders and throws a spanner in the works of biological psychiatry, because "mental disorders are profoundly different from somatic illnesses in at least one respect: many mental illnesses satisfy the externalist schema, whereas somatic illnesses do not" (Davies 2016).

He characterizes the biomedical approach to psychiatry as the view that

> the nature of mental illness is exhausted by neurological properties and events, and all facts about such conditions are scrutable from neural facts. The biomedical model also implies internalism about psychiatric disorders: features of the subject's neurophysiology suffice to determine whether or not she has a particular mental illness.
>
> (Davies 2016, 291)

We have already seen that in classifying particular disorders, both psychiatry and somatic medicine are externalist in that they sometimes depend on aetiology. But what about the decision whether a condition – which may have been classified partially by its aetiology, as in the case of PTSD – counts as pathological in the first place? Is that dependent on external factors in ways that endanger biological psychiatry and the brain disorder account?

One cannot help but feel that Davies is putting forward a bit of a straw-man characterization of the biomedical approach here. While being able to read the disorder off the neurophysiology may be a long-term goal, it is not something that people are currently proposing, let alone using as a way of identifying the presence of a certain mental disorder. Furthermore, it's been established that possible biomarkers or brain-signatures will not replace the criterion of mental dysfunction in my inclusive account of brain disorders.

Nevertheless, there is an interesting question here, which is whether we need to be able to locate some kind of difference in the brain when we distinguish between pathological and non-pathological states. The core of Davies' externalist argument against biomedical psychiatry relies on the claim that the same state looked at internalistically can be pathological or not, depending on whether it constitutes an appropriate reaction to certain external stimuli. In other words, looking at the symptoms and the brain is not enough to tell you whether a person is disordered. Davies argues that – given the criterion that low mood needs to be disproportionate – it will sometimes be impossible to distinguish sadness from depression if we do not make reference to context. According to Davies, a pathological state, depression, is distinguished from sadness by the fact that, unlike sadness, it is not warranted by the circumstances. "Given a suitably dystopian context, devoid of any reason to be happy, even the severest depressed mood might not qualify as pathological" (Davies 2016, 293). Psychiatric externalism is supposedly analogous to content externalism in that pathology 'isn't in the head'.[5] One and the same state of despair might either be perfectly warranted or pathological, depending on the state of the external world.

This kind of claim needs to be distinguished from another way in which the status of certain phenomena as pathological can be context dependent. Mental disorder diagnoses can be culturally relative in the sense that what is diagnosed as pathological in one cultural context might be considered within the realm of normal variation in another. While there obviously is cultural variation in what is considered a disorder, this is not what is at stake. It is in principle conceivable that we could all agree on what counts as a proportionate response to life events. Then there would be no cultural relativity, but there would still be context dependence in that one and the same set of psychological states can count as disordered if there are no appropriate causes but not otherwise. (If Davies is indeed correct that the decision on pathology is purely dependent on context.)

So what are we to make of the claim that we can have individuals who are impossible to distinguish if we just look at their beliefs and emotions (or, indeed, their brain states), one of whom is disordered whereas the other isn't? There are two responses I want to make. First, I want to deny that mental disorders are as disanalogous to somatic disorders as Davies suggests. Glackin (2017) has argued that in somatic disorders, too, externalist criteria decide whether a certain phenomenon counts as pathological. In as far as externalism is a feature of all medicine, it poses no special threat to brain disorder accounts of mental illness.

However, even if we pursue this strategy, there might still be some fundamental differences between somatic conditions and psychiatric ones as described by Davies. So I will also refute the strong externalism posited by Davies regarding what makes psychological states pathological. In other words, we should accept a more internalist characterization of mental disorders than that suggested by Davies. A word of reassurance for those who think that these two strategies, arguing for more externalism *and* more internalism, are contradictory. I concede that external factors play a key role in our assessment of certain states or processes as pathological. But I deny that there are no internal distinguishing features at all between those states and processes that we label as pathological and those that we don't.

3.2 Externalist somatic disorders

The claim that psychiatric disorders are fundamentally different from somatic ones due to the role externalism plays in classifying a condition as disordered has not gone unquestioned. Glackin (2017) disputes this disanalogy and argues that in somatic conditions, too, the interaction between the body and the external world is often key in characterizing a certain condition or symptom as pathological. He draws the analogy between depression and photophobia. Glackin argues that just as depression is pathological because it is a disproportionate reaction to life events, photophobia is pathological because it is a disproportionate reaction to certain light stimuli.

> Photophobia, an excessive sensitivity to or intolerance of light, can be a symptom of many conditions. Squinting or feeling discomfort is a perfectly healthy reaction to very bright light; what differentiates photophobia as pathological is that the same response is elicited by light of normal or everyday brightness. In other words, photophobia specifically involves a disproportionate or unwarranted reaction to events in the patient's environment (WHO 2016: H53.1).
> (Glackin 2017, 290)

Has Glackin given us a successful refutation of Davies' claim that psychiatric illness is externalist in a way that somatic illness is not? On one level, he has. In the photophobia example, he shows that certain external conditions are essential to categorizing certain physical reactions as pathological. But there is also an important disanalogy between photophobia and depression. In photophobia, there is an underlying physiological cause for the disproportionate reaction to light. This is more obvious in a second example Glackin uses, thrombophilia, a blood clotting disorder. He has this to say:

Blood should not clot under normal circumstances, and thrombophilias are a class of disorders in which it does so. But blood *should* clot when a patient is cut. So again, what distinguishes pathological from healthy clotting is the nature of certain antecedent events experienced by the patient (WHO 2016: D68.5, D68.6).

(Glackin 2017, 290)

Glackin's example shows that whether blood clotting is considered pathological depends on the way blood behaves in different contexts. So far, so externalist. But this example does not show that there is no internal difference between pathological and non-pathological cases. There is an identifiable biochemical difference between people who suffer from thrombophilia and those who don't. The NHS website on the topic lists a number of subtypes of thrombophilia which are distinguished by their biochemistry "protein C deficiency, protein S deficiency, antithrombine deficiency" (NHS 2020). So there clearly is an internal, biological difference between people with thrombophilia and those without. Furthermore, even in those cases where we don't know what the difference is, we assume there is some kind of difference in the body which underlies the different reaction. (Presumably, there is also an internal difference in the eyes of those suffering from photophobia and those just squinting at an overly bright light that underlies the different reactions.)

Glackin correctly notes that in order to classify conditions such as thrombophilia as disordered, we need to look at what the body (or a part thereof) is supposed to do in a certain environment. However, the analogy between somatic conditions and depression does not hold in one key respect. The claim Davies makes is that one and the same psychological profile can be pathological depending on whether it is an appropriate reaction to what is going on in the world around the person. By extension, if we know what kind of brain processes underlie the psychological states, their status as pathological, too, will depend on whether they are realizing mental states that are justified in light of the real-world events that elicit them, and there is no underlying difference which causes this maladaptive reaction. In other words, if we accept that pathology depends on external criteria, then it seems that one and the same brain process individuated internalistically may count as pathological in some contexts but not in others.

This is relevantly different from the cases that Glackin describes. *That* thrombophilia is classified as a disorder depends on how blood should behave in different circumstances. But once we have figured out the physiological causes of the specific blood clotting behaviour, we can tell whether somebody has the disorder just by looking at the physiology. By contrast, Davies claims that there is no internal psychological or physiological difference between the depressed and the justifiably sad. We might think that Davies is looking for the difference in the wrong place. In analogy to blood clotting conditions, there may be further facts which explain why, just as blood does not clot in the conditions that it should, we feel sadness or fear in situations where we shouldn't. The fact that the psychological states are supposedly indistinguishable other than by considering appropriateness conditions does not mean that there aren't further psychological or brain differences which explain why people don't behave appropriately.

It is only if there is no underlying psychological or brain difference at all that the condition is purely externalist in the way Davies requires to show a fundamental difference between mental and somatic illness. This is indeed a radically externalist scenario. Mental illness and brain pathology, too, become dependent on the relationship between the mental states they realize and the environmental stimuli when we supposedly don't even have an underlying (physiological or psychological) difference which explains the inappropriate reaction in certain circumstances. If this is indeed the situation, then Davies has a case. But as Glackin's examples show, the mere (supposed) fact that there are qualitatively identical states and processes occurring in grief and depression does not show that there is no further difference which explains the occurrence of psychological states when they are inappropriate to the stimulus. I will now cast doubt on the further hypothesis that these states are indeed qualitatively identical.

3.3 Defending limited internalism

I now want to have a closer look at the key assumption that disordered and non-disordered mental (and underlying brain) states and processes are internally indistinguishable. Does psychiatry distinguish the clinically depressed from the merely sad *exclusively* by appeal to external factors such as appropriateness considerations? The most recent DSM5 dedicates some space to drawing that very distinction. The authors of the DSM point to the fact that in grief, the predominant emotions are feelings of emptiness and loss, while in depression there is an inability to anticipate happiness or pleasure. They further note that depression is associated with feelings of guilt and worthlessness, whereas there are normally no generalized problems with self-esteem in grief (APA 2013, 161). I cannot adjudicate here whether it will be possible to draw a line reliably in all cases of depression-like sadness. But there are more differences in the phenomenology of depression and grief than Davies recognizes. This means that the claim that there is no phenomenological difference between depression and grief is inaccurate, at least if we take the diagnostic manuals seriously.

Interestingly, a similar case regarding the lack of a distinction between psychological states that we characterize as pathological and those that we don't have been made for a different disorder, addiction: neuroscientist Marc Lewis has argued that the brain changes seen in addiction are of the same kind as brain changes seen in other kinds of reinforcement learning in response to highly rewarding stimuli. "'Addiction' doesn't fit a unique physiological stamp. It simply describes the repeated pursuit of highly attractive goals and the brain changes that condense this cycle of thought and behavior into a well-learned habit" (Lewis 2017, 12).

If we believe Lewis, there is no in principle distinction between addiction and being in love in terms of cravings and the underlying brain changes. Lewis (2017) claims that we get similar dopamine release in the nucleus accumbens in addiction as we get in the process of falling in love, concluding that "if addiction is a disease, so apparently is love" (12). Looking back at the pangs of unrequited love and the urge to call the object of our desire at two in the morning, making a fool of ourselves, this may not seem that far-fetched a conclusion to draw.

However, the field is far from settled. Addiction is a condition for which the brain disorder view has been defended (but also hotly contested) for some time (Goldberg 2020). The NIDA (National Institute of Drug Abuse) lists the basal ganglia, the extended amygdala and the prefrontal cortex as brain areas affected by drug use, and also states that drug abuse leads to dopamine dysregulation (NIDA 2020). Once again, the assertion that there are not psychological or physiological differences should be taken with a grain of salt, because in places, Lewis himself talks about differences in degree, rather than kind. And in a response piece, Kent Berridge holds that the cravings we see in addiction are of such a difference in degree to other desires that they are justifiably called pathological (Berridge 2017).

What these two examples, depression and addiction, show is that claims regarding the lack of an internal difference are in need of further empirical support. In light of the current evidence, the claim that there is no difference in the mind/brain, internalistically considered, is overstated. Furthermore, the fact that we draw on the organism/environment interaction in classifying certain processes as dysfunctional does not show that there is no internal difference between states we classify as pathological and those we don't.

While I have not pursued this theoretical option here, it is worth noting that even if strong externalism were true, this would not constitute an argument against reduction. Theoretically it would be an option that mental disorders are quite different from many other somatic conditions and that one and the same brain state can count as disordered depending on context. I have not pursued this line of thought further because the arguments above are sufficient to dismantle the externalist threat as posed by Davies. One last theoretical option worth pointing out is that we can deny that conditions like addiction are disorders at all if we think there is no difference between addicted states and other strong desires. This is indeed the conclusion Lewis (2017) himself reaches. His conclusion from this supposed lack of difference between addiction and other forms of reward sensitivity and seeking is not that addiction isn't a brain disease, but that it isn't a disease at all. As a claim about how (at least some) neuroscientists and psychiatrists think about mental health conditions, the strong externalist claim seems incorrect. Rather, psychiatrists are tempted to revise the ascription of disorder if it turns out that certain conditions involve mental and brain processes that are qualitatively identical to ones that we classify as healthy.

4 Conclusion

In this chapter, I have considered two objections to my account. One objects to reduction, the other claims that externalism poses a problem for biological psychiatry. The reductionist agenda inherent in the claim that mental disorders are brain disorders need not be problematic. While my view aims at explanatory reduction, it does not imply a reductionism according to which there is a single cause in the brain that leads to the mental health condition. The worry that mental disorders cannot be reduced because of the relevance of content to mental disorder diagnoses turns out to be misguided, as it is patterns of belief or emotion rather than specific isolated contents that characterize a condition as pathological. Regarding the externalism objection, many forms of externalism are shared across somatic and psychiatric disorders. Furthermore, the claim that there are no internal psychological (or brain) differences between pathological and non-pathological phenomena such as depression and grief or addiction and other forms of reward seeking requires further empirical support.

Notes

1 I thank an anonymous reviewer for encouraging me to spell out the full ambition of the paper more clearly.
2 In their recent book on the bio-psycho-social model of health and disease, Bolton and Gillet put significant effort into showing that biological and

psychological processes and causes cannot be eliminated. They start out by pointing out that there are causal processes at the level of the biological. These are different from those in physics and chemistry in that they involve talk of purposes, aims and errors. Biology is a thoroughly normative discipline, according to them, so once we see that the laws of biology are fundamentally different to those of physics, we also see that they cannot be eliminated in favour of explanations in the terms and laws of physics. Bolton and Gillet therefore hold that the bio-psycho-social model is not compatible with physicalism, as physicalism wants to explain all causality as basically the causality of physics (57). As mentioned above, this is a rather non-standard reading both of physicalism and of reductionism. Furthermore, their project is orthogonal to the one normally ascribed to biological psychiatry, as there the reduction is *not* supposed to go all the way down to physics, but at most to mechanisms in the brain.

3 Compare (Bickle 2010), who also points out that reduction and multiple realization are not incompatible.

4 Interestingly, in the case of descriptions and explanations of delusion formation, we even have prominent accounts that are no longer clearly identifiable as being purely psychological or purely brain centred, in the form of predictive processing accounts (Corlett 2018).

5 Hilary Putnam famously argued that it is not just the descriptive content associated with a certain term that determines its reference, but also external factors such as what substance in the world we have been referring to when acquiring the term. So, when a person in the 1700s says 'water', he refers to the clear, odourless liquid which is found in the local lakes and rivers. Even though the person will at that point in history not be aware of the chemical constitution of water, H_2O, their term water refers to H_2O. Thus, if they arrive on twin earth and encounter a clear odourless liquid that looks just like the water at home but has a different chemical constitution (XYZ), they would be wrong to say that this liquid is water. The reference of a term is not just determined by the descriptive content associated with that term, but by the causal relationship between the actual substance and our linguistic practices. As Putnam memorably put it, meaning isn't in the head (Putnam 1975). Similarly, Davies tells us that pathology or dysfunction isn't in the head: just as an internal state (such as for example descriptive beliefs about a certain substance) is not enough to fix the reference of the concept WATER, symptoms of low mood alone will not be enough to establish that a person is suffering from mental illness.

5 Implications for agency and responsibility

1 Introduction

I have proposed an account of mental disorders as brain disorders according to which mental disorders are brain disorders if they are realized by systematic brain differences. We have seen that this account is reductionist, but not in the problematic way of presupposing a single aetiological brain pathway that some writers assume. We have also seen that the account is compatible with some measure of externalism, in that the interaction between individual and environment can be crucial for the status of a condition as a disorder. It is however internalist in that it posits an internal difference that leads to problematic agent/environment interactions.

But people have also argued that whether a condition is a brain disorder has effects on the agency of the person suffering from the condition, and that they are less responsible for their actions. In the case of addiction, the claim about reduced responsibility or lack of responsibility can also extend to responsibility for suffering from the condition in the first place. There are two important questions regarding how brain disorder affects agency and responsibility that I consider in this chapter. The first is whether brain disorders undermine a person's agency and responsibility *by their very nature*. Many believe this is true of mental disorders more generally, such as for example schizophrenia, but the intuition seems to be particularly strong when there is evidence of brain pathology. If it were the case that brain disorders undermine agency in some special way, this would be potentially relevant for treatment decisions, assessments of cognitive and decision making capacity, and for the assignment of moral and criminal culpability. In the context of criminal responsibility in particular, there has been an ongoing debate regarding the relevance of brain findings for individuals' *mens rea* in the context of the criminal insanity defence (Sinnott-Armstrong et al. 2008, Morse

DOI: 10.4324/9780367822088-5

2011b, 2017, Hirstein, Sifferd, and Fagan 2018). The second question concerns the effects of psychiatric labels on individuals' agency. Many worry that, irrespective of any possible effects that a condition may or may not have on agency directly, the act of *labelling* a condition as a brain disorder undermines the agency of people with that condition because of the way they themselves and others perceive them. So the first question is what implications a condition's being a brain disorder has for agency and responsibility. The second, on the other hand, focuses on the implications that the brain disorder *label* has for people.

I address these issues in turn. In Section 2, I argue that while brain pathology is relevant to agency and responsibility, judgements of responsibility focus on *psychological capacities* necessary to agency and decision making such as reasoning, perception of reality and impulse control. In our assessments of moral and legal culpability, brain pathology therefore plays at most a supporting role, giving us further information on what we really care about – psychological capacity. It can provide evidence and explanation for psychological problems that may undermine responsibility for specific actions by making it harder for the agent to recognize reasons for action or follow through on these reasons. Brain data play a far more important role in assessing an individual's capacity for some conditions than for others.

In Section 3 of this chapter, I explain why the concern about labelling effects is still worth taking seriously even though my account does not imply that brain disorders pose special additional problems to agency or responsibility. However, taking labelling effects seriously should not stop us from using the brain disorder label. While negative effects from the label 'brain disorder' or indeed descriptions or explanations of psychiatric disorders that mention brain dysfunction can arise, empirical findings on this are mixed. Furthermore, the negative effects frequently arise from various mistaken assumptions that I will outline and suggest correctives for. As labelling effects involve many individuals and institutions, it would be naive to think there is an easy fix for them where they do arise. Nevertheless, it is possible to give some pointers as to how further improvement is possible.

2 Do brain disorders undermine agency and responsibility?

Psychological capacities are of central importance for agency and responsibility, both looking forward and looking backward, and mental disorders can undermine a person's legal right to make their own decisions, but also their criminal culpability for wrongful behaviour. For example, the United Kingdom's mental capacity act of 2005 lays down conditions under which a person is deemed to be unable to make their own decisions:

> a person lacks capacity in relation to a matter if at the material time he is unable to make a decision for himself in relation to the matter because of an impairment of, or a disturbance in the functioning of, the mind or brain.

(2005C9, 2.1)

If a person is deemed to lack mental capacity in a certain area, they will not be allowed to make certain decisions, for example financial decisions like buying or selling a house for themselves. Loss of mental capacity may affect only the right to specific types of decisions and is often reversible. The way mental disorders affect decision making is also important in backward looking criminal contexts: if a person is thought not to be able to understand the nature and wrongfulness of their action, they may be excused from criminal culpability through the insanity defence.

There is a widespread belief that if someone suffers from brain pathology, then this implies that their actions are not responsive to reasons and they are not responsible for their actions. In this vein, Szasz criticizes the view that mental disorders are brain disorders as "the image of the patients as the helpless victims of pathobiological events outside their control" (Szasz 2011, 179). Similarly, Arpaly (2005) points to a common set of assumptions: when we describe a condition like, for example, depression as 'a chemical imbalance in the brain', this often goes hand in hand with viewing the actions of a person suffering from depression as caused by brute mechanical forces, rather than by reasoning processes we recognize and can interpret as responsive to reasons for action. Just as fractious behaviour in tired small children is often ascribed to their tiredness and not as a response to what the child is ostensibly getting upset about, the behaviour of those suffering from depression is sometimes ascribed to the depression. The extent to which reasoning and decision making capacities are affected by mental disorders generally and brain pathology in particular is relevant both to forward looking aspects of agency (what decisions can the person competently make, do they have mental capacity) and to ascribing responsibility in a backward looking way, in particular when it comes to moral and legal culpability. As there is insufficient space to discuss in detail how cognitive capacities are affected in both the forward looking and the backward looking cases, I will focus on moral and criminal culpability in the following.

The relevance of brain pathology to issues of culpability has been a subject of lively debate in this millennium (Morse 2011a, Farahany 2016).

The tendency to think someone is not responsible is more marked if a condition like, for example, schizophrenia is conceptualized as a brain disorder. Our intuitions on this topic are a tangled mess. I will discuss people's perceptions of how brain disorder affects responsibility and agency in the section on labelling below. But first, here is how we *should* think about the relationship between mental disorder, brain dysfunction, and agency and responsibility: responsible agency requires certain reasoning and decision making capacities. We need to be able to evaluate reasons for action, and we need at least some measure of impulse control. In the literature on moral responsibility, this is called reasons-responsiveness. Reasons-responsiveness requires both the ability to recognize reasons to act (or not to act) in a certain way and the ability to actually act on these reasons at least some of the time (Fischer and Ravizza 1998). Reasons-responsiveness is a notion which was first developed in order to specify compatibilist conditions on moral responsibility for all humans to show how we can be morally responsible even if determinism is true.

Another way to specify the conditions for responsibility is that we need two capacities. First, we need to fulfil an epistemic condition (reasons receptivity in Fischer and Ravizza's account): we need to understand the moral character of our actions. We also need some level of control over the way we decide and act (reasons reactivity). Whether someone has the requisite control for moral responsibility is normally spelled out by asking whether they would act in the way that is morally required in fairly similar scenarios. So, for example, Lucy is considered to have the requisite control not to steal (even if she does sometimes steal) if she refrains from stealing in situations where there is a shop detective nearby, when she knows she is likely to be caught, or if she has been reminded of the immorality of stealing recently. Exactly how to assess the degree of control an agent has is notoriously difficult.

In as far as a psychiatric illness and associated brain dysfunction undermines these capacities for understanding the morality of one's actions and controlling them, it also undermines responsibility. The impact of a psychiatric disorder on these capacities may also vary depending upon specific situations and over time (King and May 2018). Given that moral responsibility is concerned with these psychological capacities, for all practical purposes, the importance of brain dysfunction is evidential. Knowing about certain processes in the brain will help us evaluate the psychological capacities relevant to responsible agency. Information relating to the brain will vary a lot in how much it tells us about psychological capacities. In many cases, behavioural evidence will be primary, for example when we ask about impulse control, as in the above stealing cases. The ability to control one's impulses is defined through a behavioural profile across situations and incentivization scenarios. We can then investigate what brain anomalies are associated with anomalies in impulse control. In other cases, brain data will be extremely relevant in telling us about psychological capacities. For example, fMRI data help distinguish between patients with locked in syndrome and coma, a distinction that is hard to draw on behavioural evidence (Heinrichs 2019, 216). While this is not a case where the question of moral and criminal responsibility arises, given the inability to act, it illustrates the importance brain data can have in informing us about (the existence of) psychological states.

So, what matters to agency and responsibility – be it moral or legal – is the way certain psychological processes are affected by a psychiatric condition. This means that when we assess whether a condition undermines a person's agency, brain data are relevant only in as far as they can be translated into the psychological capacities central to being a responsible agent. If a condition undermines reasons-responsiveness because it leads to severely impaired impulse control or an inability to assess the rightness of one's action, it will affect a person's moral responsibility. An inability to assess the rightness of one's action may arise through delusional beliefs that make actions seem reasonable and even moral when in fact they are not. A famous example of this is the case of Andrea Yates, who drowned her children, because she believed this would save them from Satan (Associated Press 2006, Morse 2008). Yates was suffering from post-partum psychosis, and her delusional beliefs affected her ability to judge the rightness of her action. Judgements of responsibility should be made on the basis of psychological features of the agent, not primarily on the basis of brain findings (Vincent 2008, Morse 2011b, 2017, Jefferson 2022).

The fact that in making judgements of agency and responsibility we focus on a person's psychological capacities does not mean that brain findings are irrelevant to such judgements. If we understand the way in which the brain realizes reasons-responsiveness, brain findings can corroborate, or even explain, certain psychological findings regarding a person's moral agency. When specific brain differences are found that underlie specific psychological deviations from the norm, this may indicate that a person's moral agency is compromised. Spelling out the exact way in which brain findings would support the lack of relevant psychological capacities is beyond the scope of this book, and there are competing accounts, depending on what psychological features are thought essential for reasons-responsiveness. For example, Bill Hirstein, Katrina Sifferd and Ty Fagan have recently argued that executive function is crucial to having the mental capacities necessary for responsible agency and reasons-responsiveness, and that executive function is impaired in many mental disorders (Hirstein, Sifferd, and Fagan 2018). The term 'executive function' refers to a set of cognitive processes such as working memory, response inhibition, selective attention and cognitive flexibility. Impairment of executive function, they argue, is measurable at the level of the brain, as there are a number of networks in the brain that have been identified as subserving executive function. Thus, they establish a link between brain dysfunction and moral responsibility via problems with executive function. By contrast, Neil Levy argues that certain emotional capacities are key to responsible agency, as they correct individuals' ability to realize the wrongness of harming others (Levy 2007). Thus, whether individuals suffering from a mental disorder are morally and legally responsible for a specific wrongful action depends on whether any brain disorder they may have significantly impacts psychological capacities necessary for responsibility.

So, brain dysfunction and disorder are important for agency and responsibility, but they inform our responsibility judgements indirectly, by telling us more about the psychological capacities an individual has. In addition to cases where brain dysfunction realizes psychological dysfunction, there are also cases of paradigmatic brain disorders where there is a clear causal link between brain pathology, lack of impulse control and problematic behaviour. This has been observed in patients with brain tumours (Burns and Swerdlow 2003, Lipska 2018) and in some cases of fronto-temporal dementia (Pompanin et al. 2014). However, even in these cases, we need to look at the behavioural evidence when it comes to assessing agency and responsibility. We cannot jump straight from the fact that there is brain pathology to the assumption that agency is compromised (Morse 2011b, Jefferson 2022), but we need to look at the extent to which the person affected shows control problems more generally.

This issue has been discussed in detail regarding the case study of a man who developed paedophilic urges because of a brain tumour and started behaving inappropriately, collecting child pornography and eventually making advances on his young step-daughter. Over time, his behaviour became ever more erratic and a brain tumour was discovered. The tumour clearly played a crucial causal role in the man's behaviour: once the man's tumour was operated upon, the paedophilic urges went away, the man's behaviour returned to normal and he was able to return to his family (Burns and Swerdlow 2003). It may be tempting to think that the special causal role the tumour played means that it deprived him of agency and excused the man's behaviour. This is indeed the line of reasoning we see in Moncrieff, who compares cases like the brain tumour with epilepsy and claims that pedophilic behaviour is not attributable to the individual's agency but to their disease (Moncrieff 2020, 174).

However, Awais Aftab points out that this comparison is not apt – paedophilic behaviour, unlike epileptic fits, "does involve conscious awareness and decision-making" (Aftab 2020, 318). This means that we still need to assess the individual's psychological capacities in order to assess their responsibility. As Morse (2011b) argues, and I concur, we cannot just move from the fact that a tumour *caused* the paedophilic urges to the conclusion that the man lacked control and was not responsible, but need to look at the behavioural evidence more generally. The behavioural evidence in this specific case suggests that the man did not have control over his behaviour shortly before the tumour was finally discovered, because he was acting in erratic and impulsive ways that were clearly at odds with his own self-interest. However, matters are less clearly cut in the early stages of his illness when he started collecting child pornography and hiding the evidence from his family and making advances on his step-daughter.

One might object that severe brain pathology should automatically provide an excuse in this kind of case, because of the way problems with impulse control or moral understanding come about. The man unexpectedly developed these urges through no fault of his own. I am somewhat sympathetic to this line of reasoning as I believe that sudden changes to our psychology, be they caused by mental illness or a tumour, may leave us with strong urges, strong emotions or strange beliefs for which we do not have coping mechanisms (Jefferson 2022). But in as far as this provides an excuse, the excuse stems from the sudden, unexpected changes in our psychology, rather than from the fact that this is a case of brain pathology.

To summarize, while brain dysfunction often *does* matter to moral responsibility and agency, there is no automatic inference from 'suffers from brain dysfunction' to 'has reduced agency and responsibility'. Rather, we need to look at the way an individual reasons and acts and listen to the way they explain and evaluate their actions in order to assess the extent to which their agency is compromised. We can then assess whether the agent is responsible in light of our theory specifying the mental capacities necessary for responsibility and agency. To do otherwise would be disrespectful and stigmatizing: it would be an approach where we jump to the conclusion that a person's behaviour does not make sense on the basis of a diagnosis alone (Arpaly 2005, Broome, Bortolotti, and Mameli 2010, Jeppsson 2021).

3 Labelling effects

So far, I have been concerned with the question whether, and if so how, brain disorders undermine agency and responsibility. However, one might concede everything I have said and still be worried about applying the term 'brain disorder' in the way I propose. Why is this? The essence of this worry is that, irrespective of how the term brain disorder *should* best be understood, it is in practice understood in ways that are detrimental to the people labelled as suffering from a brain disorder. One important concern is that brain disorder labels undermine agency through people's *belief* that brain disorders are bodily conditions that override an individual's agency and decision making, leaving them a helpless victim to 'what their brain makes them do'. We have already seen in the previous section that this is not the right way of thinking of brain disorders and dysfunctions. But, if it is what people in fact think, it is still a problem. As I argue elsewhere, perception matters: if we believe certain actions and decisions lie outside our power, then we will not even attempt them (Jefferson 2020a). In what follows, I will argue that while the 'brain disorder' label can have negative effects, the empirical picture is mixed. Furthermore, there are things we can and should do to reduce stigma and misperceptions of the implications of brain dysfunction.

Thus, discussions about diagnostic labels do not just revolve around the question whether there are good theoretical reasons not to classify an x as a y. Rather, people worry about the practical effects of such a diagnosis and whether it does more harm than good. Irrespective of its theoretical adequacy, a diagnostic category shapes reality and produces an interactive kind if it is commonly used. When we evaluate labelling, or a categorization, one of the things we check is whether the label has been used correctly. Labels can be accurate or inaccurate; we can mislabel something in very straightforward ways. If you buy a packet of tablets which says 'Aspirin' on the pack and upon opening them, you find that the packet in fact contains paracetamol, this is a case of mislabelling. Similarly, though more controversially, you can diagnose someone as having unipolar depression when in fact they are suffering from bipolar disorder. That kind of case is more controversial because experts disagree about psychiatry's diagnostic labels themselves. One of the crucial questions in psychiatry and clinical psychology is not just whether I was right in labelling Mia as schizophrenic, but whether the label 'schizophrenia' picks out a genuine pattern in the world or, in the terms of the trade, whether it's a valid diagnostic category or construct (Huda 2019, 93). Diagnostic constructs can be valid or not.

Apart from judging its validity, we can also evaluate a diagnostic category for its effects. Diagnostic labels in psychiatry are infamous for not just describing reality but shaping it. Mental health conditions are one of philosopher Ian Hacking's primary examples of interactive or looping kinds. For example, he argues that an autism diagnosis does not just give information about an independently existing condition, but also shapes what being autistic is through the way experts, institutions, people diagnosed as autistic and their friends and family perceive and understand the condition. The autism diagnosis and the way people interact with it create 'a different way of being a person'. Practitioners, individuals diagnosed and society more generally develop a body of information and beliefs about a condition which feeds back into a diagnostic category and the model of the condition. This is particularly striking in the case of autism, both in terms of the ever-growing proportion of the population diagnosed as autistic, the current trend towards self-diagnosis, and the movement to re-conceptualize autism as a form of neurodiversity rather than as a disorder. Hacking calls the way in which people interacting with a diagnostic category changes that category itself the 'looping effect' (Hacking 2007, 2009).

The fact that labels change people's way of being in the world raises moral questions, and there is significant evidence that diagnostic labels are stigmatizing (Corrigan 2007, Parcesepe and Cabassa 2013). Adverse effects of labels are frequently used as an objection against certain diagnostic categories. For example, the 'drop the disorder' movement holds that we should get rid of psychiatric diagnoses altogether (Watson 2019). As one would expect, use of the brain disorder label is hotly contested: it has been employed both in an effort to destigmatize mental health conditions (Leshner 1997, Malla, Joober, and Garcia 2015) and criticized for increasing stigma (Hart 2017, Satel and Lilienfeld 2017). This debate has been particularly virulent in the context of addiction. Some clinicians and researchers claim that labelling certain conditions as brain disorders has detrimental effects on the people labelled as having that condition. For example, Sally Satel and Scott Lilienfeld (2017) argue that labelling addiction as a brain disorder undermines treatment success, as people will then think of addiction as a brute mechanical process that overrides rational decision making, because it is a disorder of the body. According to their argument, the label thereby entrenches addiction. Furthermore, in the wilds of Twitter, we find claims that the brain disorder label is purely instrumental, a drug selling ploy by big pharma.

As it happens, many critics of the brain disorder label think it is both theoretically inadequate and practically pernicious. Furthermore, even theoretically inadequate labels can create real patterns in the way conditions manifest if Hacking is correct about interactive kinds: you can create kinds even if the diagnostic construct you employ is not a valid one. As I understand it, this is what Hacking thinks happened with the diagnostic category 'multiple personality disorder', which flourished for a while and heavily influenced the symptoms people presented with. The number of alters (different personalities) a person presented with increased, and there was an increased (possibly inaccurate) recall of childhood abuse. When the diagnostic category was changed to dissociative identity disorder, this also came with a change in symptoms and a different way of being. According to Hacking, "[The new label] was no mere change in name, no mere act of diagnostic house-cleaning. Symptoms evolve, patients are no longer expected to come with a roster of altogether distinct personalities, and they no longer do" (Hacking 2007, 300).[1] As I understand it, kinds are, at least in part, created by labelling processes. This creates the possibility of having a diagnostic category that does not pick out what it purports to pick out, but still shapes reality. Clearly, this is not the scenario I am worried about regarding the concept of brain disorder I put forward. I am convinced of its theoretical adequacy and have tried to persuade you, dear reader, of it as well. But there is another problematic constellation: in principle, one can have a perfectly theoretically sound category of classification which still has undesirable effects on people's self-perception or the way others see them. This is the worry I address here.

Desirability and undesirability of diagnostic labels is a feature that is in principle separable from diagnostic accuracy and arises from the way people react to the diagnosis. Undesirability of diagnostic labels stems from the effects they have on people, primarily the people diagnosed as having a condition. When people receive a diagnosis, they start to see themselves in a different light. For example, a study by Crystal Hoyt and colleagues (2014) looked at the influence that labelling obesity as a disease had on obese study participants. They found that after hearing the message, people felt better about themselves but they were also less likely to attach importance to healthy food choices and more likely to choose high calorie foods. These kinds of effects on people's perceptions and actions are the reason why desirability plays such a strong role in arguments for and against a certain diagnostic category. Clinicians and researchers worry about the way a category will affect the self-image of people categorized, but also whether they will be stigmatized by others. But practical ramifications extend beyond stigma: on a level of policy, neuroscientist Carl Hart argues that labelling drug addiction as a brain disease comes at a significant cost for intervention and treatment, because it focuses attention on the drug-brain interaction to the exclusion of social and economic factors driving drug use in certain communities. What we call something and the theoretical model people associate with the label will significantly affect how what is labelled manifests itself.

The brain disorder label is a way of classifying health conditions, but it is not a diagnostic category in the way say 'schizophrenia' or 'depression' is. Rather, the label subsumes many different conditions, mental health conditions (at least on some accounts) as well as conditions such as Parkinson's or stroke. If this label indeed has the negative effects some authors propose, this is a problem that needs to be taken seriously. However, in as far as people draw conclusions that are not justified by the category and the theory associated with it, the correct move is to try to influence people's understanding of the label, rather than abandoning it. Furthermore, scientists have endorsed classifying a condition as a brain disorder on the reasoning that this would have positive, destigmatizing effects.

When people predict or postulate certain effects, they are frequently heavily influenced by the model of the phenomenon they themselves endorse. They think a specific theoretical model *implies* certain practical consequences, and may even be endorsing a theoretical model because of its perceived practical implications. We can see this in the debate about whether addiction or schizophrenia are brain disorders. In his landmark paper, Alan Leshner (1997) famously argued that 'addiction is a brain disease and it matters'. His contention was that conceptualizing addiction as a brain disease is scientifically correct because addiction involves specific pathological changes in brain activity and structure. It is also desirable because it diminishes blame of addicts which arises when people view addiction merely as a bad habit or a moral failing. Leshner hopes that, once we come to see that there is something wrong with the brains of people suffering from addiction, we will become less judgemental towards them.

Conversely, Satel and Lilienfeld argue against the addiction as brain disease view by pointing out all the differences to classic brain diseases such as brain tumours. This is an objection to the correctness of using that term. They also object that people do not take responsibility for their drug taking behaviour because they see it as determined by a purely physiological process. This is a claim about the undesirability of using the term. A similar strategy is pursued by Carl Hart, who argues that if we think of addiction as primarily about the interaction between the brain and the addictive substance, we will ignore important social factors (Hart 2017).

While this approach to predicting effects of the use of a certain label on stigma, treatment etc. is understandable, it disregards the fact that in the real world, others do not endorse the model we ourselves endorse and may associate the same term with a different model. We have already seen that this is the case for the term 'brain disorder'. So, I can't really use my own model to predict effects, and neither can people with other, different models. If we want to know whether practical consequences such as decreased sense of agency or increased stigma are indeed a consequence of calling a condition a brain disorder, we need to review empirical findings on the associations people in fact have with these labels.

3.1 Empirical findings

In order to make a judgement regarding the positive or negative effects of a diagnosis, we first need to establish what these effects are. There is, at this stage, a substantial body of research concerning people's associations with diagnostic labels generally and labelling a condition a brain disorder in particular. In the context of schizophrenia, Corrigan and Watson (2004) hypothesize that labelling schizophrenia a brain disorder may lead to mixed benefits. It may reduce the perception that the condition is somehow the fault of the people who have it, but increase perceptions of dangerousness and otherness, and also make people more ready to assume that the condition is permanent and immutable.

> People make attributions about not only the onset of a disorder (Is schizophrenia caused by weak character or biology?) but also its offset (Will the person get better so he or she can live a normal life?). Framing mental illness as a brain disorder may resolve onset questions but exacerbate offset issues.
> (Corrigan and Watson 2004, 477)

Research on the effects of diagnostic labels does not always come readily packaged for the purposes of this chapter, often it does not look at associations with the term 'brain disorder' specifically. Where it does, the research frequently explicitly posits a biological aetiology, biological risk factors or neuroscientific explanations of symptoms or the aetiology of the condition. While these kinds of factors are compatible with the brain disorder account I put forward, most of them only pick out a subset of the conditions my account would label as brain disorders, as they are once again focused on aetiology, rather than realization. But we have to work with the material that is available.

Meta-analyses found that while biogenetic explanations of psychiatric conditions were associated with decreased blaming responses, they increased perceptions of dangerousness and desire for social distance (Kvaale, Gottdiener, and Haslam 2013, Kvaale, Haslam, and Gottdiener 2013). A more recent meta-analysis compiled the findings regarding the relationship between specifically *neuroscientific* explanations of mental disorder and stigmatizing beliefs across several studies. The authors note that one might reasonably expect a difference in reaction to biogenetic explanations and to neuroscientific explanations. They hypothesize that people see biogenetic explanations, especially genetic ones, as essentialist in a way they might not do for brain-centred explanations: "although laypeople may understand genes as causally potent essences that are discrete and static, they may understand brain phenomena in less binary and more dynamic ways, encouraged perhaps by popular writing on neural plasticity" (Loughman and Haslam 2018). This seems like a reasonable hypothesis, and one that would be conducive to an understanding of brain disorder that does not assume that the level of psychological treatment and conscious decision making becomes irrelevant in brain disorders.

However, the authors found that many of the associations found in earlier studies about biogenetic explanations also held when participants endorsed neuroscientific explanations: these explanations were associated with greater perceived dangerousness, a greater desire for social distance and more pessimism about the likelihood of recovery. The one difference they found was that there was no positive or negative effect for blame; endorsement of neuroscientific explanations did not affect blame negatively or positively. When looking at individual studies rather than the broad trends that meta-analyses identify, findings are mixed. For example, Miresco and Kirmayer (2006) found that brain explanations were associated with lower perceived responsibility than psychological ones. By contrast, De Brigard and colleagues did not find that describing the way a mental health problem contributed to an action in neuroscientific terms made a difference to responsibility judgements (De Brigard, Mandelbaum, and Ripley 2008).

The mixed results found in the literature are unsurprising given the level of disagreement about what exactly brain disorders are that we have seen throughout this book and indeed, in this chapter. Furthermore, the robustness of the empirical findings depends on the quality of the design of the studies that generated these findings. For example, I have methodological reservations about the study by Miresco et al., which found that clinicians were less likely to ascribe responsibility and control to people whose condition was described as resulting from brain pathology. There are likely confounding factors that the authors do not take into account. For starters, the symptoms and phenomenology of the conditions they compare (mania, heroin addiction and personality disorders) are completely different independently of any brain/mind difference. A person is very different from their usual self when in a manic phase, in a way that isn't the case for personality disorders. It is likely that this explains a lot of the variation they find. Furthermore, in the vignettes the authors present to study participants, the manic episode is medication-induced (by SSRIs) and therefore the (unintended) result of a medical intervention. This is also likely to make a difference to people's intuitions. Without probing the individual studies in detail, looking at meta-analyses can only give us a snapshot overview. Nevertheless, the summarized findings do indicate that there is a tendency to draw undesirable conclusions when told that someone is suffering from a brain disorder.

3.2 Explaining effects and counteracting them

Irrespective of how common undesirable effects of labels are, if we want to counteract them, we need to know why they arise. I will canvas two plausible explanations for undesirable effects and propose mitigation strategies that can counteract these effects.

3.2.1 Analogies and paradigms

Most lay people probably don't have a worked-out model of brain disorder when they make judgements about responsibility and agency, likely treatment success, etc. based on the information that a condition is a brain disorder or involves brain dysfunction. Rather, lay people, as well as experts, rely heavily on comparisons to paradigm cases, as I have outlined throughout the book. This may be the comparison to diabetes (Malla, Joober, and Garcia 2015), cancer (Szasz 2011, Satel and Lilienfeld 2017), or neurosyphilis (Pickard 2018, Radden 2018). So, for example, the comparison to cancer leads naturally to the idea that if something in our brain is broken it will only be fixable by interventions on the body, be these surgical or pharmaceutical. Satel and Lilienfeld point out that in a brain disease like cancer, there is nothing we can do to treat or manage the disease through our own thinking and decision making. The only thing that will help is an operation and/or chemotherapy. This is precisely why they object to using the brain disorder label to addiction, but also to understanding it in analogy to cancer. In fairness to Satel and Lilienfeld, this analogy is frequently introduced by proponents of the brain disorder view:

> No amount of reward or punishment can alter the course of, say, brain cancer. It is an entirely autonomous biological condition. Imagine threatening to impose a penalty on a brain cancer victim if her vision or speech continued to worsen or to offer of $1 million if she could stay well. It wouldn't matter.
>
> Addiction, by comparison, is a complex set of activities whose course can be altered when the user confronts foreseeable consequences.
>
> (Satel and Lilienfeld 2017)

If we take the brain disorder or dysfunction to show that the problem is of the same kind as in conditions where the problem is one of uncontrolled cell growth (cancer), cell death (Alzheimer's) or bacterial infection (neurosyphilis), this will of course have implications for the role of the individual in treatment. On this model, the psychology merely follows, while the brain breaks and gets fixed on its own. But, as we have already explored in Chapter 2, it does not follow from the fact that addiction is a brain disorder or even from the analogy to cancer that it is exactly like cancer in all respects. Analogies between different disorders or diseases are always approximate. We have also seen that even in the case of cancer, it's premature to jump to the conclusion that people are automatically not blameworthy for wrongful action in this chapter.

Does this mean we should stop using these kinds of analogies? It is not realistic or desirable to abstain from drawing analogies altogether. Reasoning by analogy is the bread and butter of much of our thinking. However, we could improve matters by drawing on a more balanced diet of analogies. For example, we can draw on paradigmatic cases of brain pathology which still require a large amount of individual effort and agency in treatment, such as for example stroke. While stroke is a classic case where the aetiology is clearly biological (physiological), rehabilitation from stroke is very much dependent on the patient doing exercises and taking action. Even diabetes, a clearly somatic condition that is often used in analogies between psychiatric and somatic conditions requires lifestyle changes that go well beyond taking medication for successful management. Different comparisons, such as the one with stroke, might be highlighted to show the importance of agency in the treatment of even paradigmatic brain disorders. But we also need to make the limitations of analogies very clear and explain the theoretical basis for calling a condition a brain disorder, which is that we have found dysfunction in the brain for that condition. Otherwise, there is a danger of further analogies importing further errors or reinforcing existing ones. For example, the stroke analogy invites the thought that only those conditions with a brain aetiology which can be specified independently of psychology are brain disorders. So it should be stressed that brain disorders and instances of brain dysfunction encompass a wide range of conditions which are in many ways quite different from paradigmatic brain disorders.

For example, addiction understood as a brain disorder is still quite different from paradigmatic brain disorders (on the assumption that we want to call addiction a disorder in the first place). It can develop in response to many substances, and if we accept that there are process addictions, we don't even need the substances. Furthermore, proponents of the brain disease model of addiction and the choice model of addiction agree on the fact that there are significant brain changes in addiction (Goldberg 2020). To avoid negative labelling effects, we should draw attention to how varied even paradigmatic brain disorders can be and also point out both the similarities and the important differences to the comparison cases we evoke.

3.2.2 Intuitive dualism

Even when the model of brain disorder explicitly separates itself from claims about aetiology, treatment, lack of agency, etc., old intuitions die hard. Thus, when talking about treatment for mental disorders conceived as brain disorders, Insel and Cuthbert state that "paradoxically, one of the most powerful and precise interventions to alter such activity might be targeted psychotherapy, such as cognitive behavioural therapy" (Insel and Cuthbert 2015, 500). That targeted psychotherapy should be the best approach is only paradoxical if one thinks that brain disorders are mechanical defects that arise and persist independently of psychological processes. Why are people drawn to beliefs about purely physical treatment for brain dysfunction even when they explicitly reject the underlying narrow model of brain disorder? One possible answer that has repeatedly been mooted is that people are intuitive dualists. They (the intuitive dualists) therefore think that explanations of behaviour or mental states in brain terms and explanations in mental terms are mutually exclusive. Even people who are theoretically committed to a materialist world-view supposedly think about psychiatric illness in dualist ways, thinking that if the brain is not functioning as it should, people lack agency and accountability, and need to be treated by intervention on the body. While initially appealing as an explanation, this diagnosis of intuitive dualism is deeply wrong-headed, as I explain below.

We can find the claim that people are intuitive dualists and therefore equate brain dysfunction with lack of agency espoused by various authors. Miresco and Kirmayer (2006) claim to have found dualistic thinking in psychiatrists which affected psychiatrists' perceptions of patients' agency and responsibility. (Though see my comments above on methodological issues concerning their study.) In the context of neuroscientific explanations of, for example, addictive cravings, dualistic intuitions may make us think that the existence of a pathological brain process that can be mechanistically described negates the relevance of mental reasoning and decision making processes. In a different context, Joshua Greene and Jonathan Cohen (2011) have argued that increasing knowledge of the brain processes at work in decision making will make all of us stop believing in free will and responsibility. If this is indeed the case, then the way of changing people's perceptions would go via challenging that intuition that there is a distinction between your brain processing information and your mind thinking. It is to be hoped that some change will happen naturally as people get more used to thinking about the way brain processes realize cognition.

But there is a more fundamental problem with the intuitive dualism explanation of people's reaction to the brain disorder label. If people do think that brain explanations are not compatible with intentional ones, this is a problem for our understanding of agency and responsibility in general, not just in the context of mental health. All mental processes are realized by brain processes. If intuitive dualism undermines our conception of humans as reasons-responsive creatures, it does so across the board. This is indeed the consequence Greene and Cohen draw when they argue that neuroscience will undermine our belief in free will and responsibility. If we intuitively think that brain focused explanations of decision making are incompatible with explanations of decisions as based on reasons, then there is a problem with responsible agency for all humans, not just for those with mental disorders.

But we can turn this argument on its head: if we *don't* think that brain focused descriptions of decision making pose a problem for our concept of rational decision making in general, then intuitive dualism should not automatically undermine ascriptions of intentional and reasons-responsive decision making in cases where there is brain dysfunction. The fact that we can show how dysfunctional brain processes are involved in the decisions of people suffering from mental disorder does not in itself make that decision making any less intentional or imply that there is no reasoning going on. Whether there is a problem with agency depends on how exactly the psychological dysfunction caused or realized by the brain dysfunction affects reasoning and decision-making capacities. In sum, consistency of reasoning requires us to conclude that intuitive dualism does not pose a special problem for the moral agency of people suffering from mental disorders conceived as brain disorders.

One might object that my rebuttal is too theory driven. Just because intuitive dualists should reject agency across the board, does not mean they will, because people are inconsistent in their thinking. The reason that people can combine intuitive dualism with a belief in agency is because they are not normally confronted with the way the brain is involved in thought, emotion and decision making. The focus on brain dysfunction makes brain processes more salient and triggers dualistic intuitions. The first thing to say about this is that it's an empirical hypothesis in search of empirical support. But even if the hypothesis turned out to be true, the right approach to this is not to shrug and let people continue thinking about these matters in an inconsistent fashion. If we are not worried that physicalism and neuroscientific descriptions of decision making generally undermine agency, we should not be worried about it in the context of psychiatric conditions.

It is entirely possible that certain brain dysfunctions undermine responsibility for specific actions, but if so, they do that in virtue of the way that the brain dysfunction impacts certain psychological capacities important to moral agency. It is to be hoped that as people get more used to neuroscience as part of psychology, psychiatry and medicine, they will be less inclined to think of brain processes and psychological processes as an *either/or*. So, while I think intuitive dualism is a hypothesis worth taking seriously, we should not be too pessimistic about people's ability to take a more sophisticated view. As our understanding of the brain and the way it processes information increases, it is to be hoped that our intuitions become less dualistic.

To summarize, while there is some evidence of undesirable effects of the brain disorder label, in particular on perceived agency, the likely reasons can, and should, be counteracted.

4 Conclusion

The fact that an individual suffers from a brain disorder has no *automatic* implications for agency and moral responsibility. However, brain dysfunction and the associated psychological dysfunction excuses from responsibility or mitigates it in cases where the condition affects that person's reasons-responsiveness in a certain situation. Brain findings are therefore an important further source of evidence regarding how capacities important for moral decision making and decision making more generally may be affected. It is, of course, true that brain disorder is sometimes the cause of impaired capacities, as in the case where the man acquired paedophilic tendencies because of his brain tumour. Nevertheless, it is capacities that matter for responsibility assessments.

Labelling effects may well have a negative effect on people through misperceptions of what the label implies. Beliefs about reduced agency because one is suffering from a brain disorder may sometimes become self-fulfilling. I have argued that certain models of brain disorders, unwarranted parallels to paradigm cases, and dualist intuitions may all drive these effects. Consequently, there are some things we can do to counter these effects: we should endorse and disseminate better models (i.e., mine). We should make both the analogies and the disanalogies explicit when we appeal to paradigm cases and introduce a more varied range of comparisons. Finally, we should try our best to get people to think less dualistically about the mind/brain relationship, so that they don't think of brain explanations and reason based explanations for action as mutually exclusive. Of course, given the many parties who play a role in labelling effects, any given intervention will have limited effects. But that does not mean we should not continue trying.

Note

1 Hacking largely steers clear of questions of diagnostic validity, but he does distinguish between transient disorders such as multiple personality disorders which did not exist prior to the diagnosis, and conditions such as autism, which did (Hacking 2007).

6 Conclusion

Over the course of this book, I have put forward and defended an inclusive view of brain disorders. I have shown that objections to the claim that mental disorders are brain disorders frequently arise from a narrow view of brain disorders and that my inclusive view is not vulnerable to many of the challenges that detractors of brain disorder views put forward.

On the inclusive view of brain disorders, there is more than one way of being a brain disorder. Paradigmatic brain disorders where there is a clearly identifiable aetiology in the brain are one kind of brain disorder; this is the only kind of brain disorder recognized by the narrow view. I have argued that the narrow view unnecessarily restricts the extension of the term 'brain disorder' to conditions that resemble paradigmatic brain disorders. It is also too narrowly focused on aetiology and treatment. While aetiology and treatment may provide practical grounds for distinguishing between different conditions, the narrow view cannot provide good theoretical reasons to exclude anomalies in brain function that realize dysfunctional psychological processes from the category of brain dysfunctions. Furthermore, many factors are involved in aetiology and treatment, so appeal to these two categories does not provide a clear distinction between brain disorders and purely mental disorders. It is, however, true that some disorders are more obviously 'brainy' than others, in that brain pathology is more heavily involved in the aetiology and treatment requires direct intervention on the brain through, e.g. medication.

As well as presenting and criticizing the narrow view of brain disorders, I have shown that it is still very prominent in the thinking of many people who reject the claim that mental disorders can also be brain disorders. My view also needs to be distinguished from another common view that I take to be misguided, the over-inclusive view. People who endorse the over-inclusive view believe that materialism implies that all

DOI: 10.4324/9780367822088-6

mental disorders are brain disorders, because there are no mental states and activities without the brain. This is the view that many philosophers intuitively lean towards at first pass.

The reason why this view is nevertheless over-inclusive can be found in thinking about the multiple realizability of mental states and the multi-functionality of brain areas. In order to ascribe a dysfunction, we need to identify a type of brain process that is behaving anomalously. We need both patterns of normal functioning and patterns of dysfunction. I use the plural advisedly; there can be more than one way in which the brain realizes mental dysfunction. But there cannot be endless ways. There needs to be something that brains are doing differently from the non-pathological case in order for them to be exhibiting a dysfunction. If there is no pattern of dysfunction, there is no dysfunction at the level of the brain. Here is another way of seeing this: if the brain of a healthy person is indistinguishable from that of one suffering from a mental illness, then we would have to say that one and the same type of brain process is both functional and dysfunctional. (Note that context dependence is not a way out here – we can build the context into normal functioning and say that it is the reaction of the mind or brain to a certain stimulus that we are considering.)

We thus end up with a view of brain disorder which is more inclusive than the narrow view, as it includes cases of brain dysfunction where a brain difference is realizing a psychological dysfunction. But, in contrast to the over-inclusive view, it doesn't allow any token realizer of psychological dysfunction to automatically count as dysfunctional. This view of brain disorder fits well with the RDoC's understanding of brain disorders as disorders of neural circuits.

My account is reductionist in the sense that it requires explanatory reduction in order to classify a mental disorder as a brain disorder. This reduction will take place at the level of symptoms and dysfunctional psychological processes, rather than at the level of diagnostic categories as a whole. Contrary to what critics claim, another kind of reduction, single-cause-brain-aetiology reduction, is not presupposed or required by the inclusive view of brain disorders.

Like all disorders, somatic or psychiatric, what counts as a disorder is partly determined by factors outside the agent. Certain conditions count as pathological because they involve inappropriate responses to environmental stimuli. In that respect, mental disorders are externalist. However, I reject the claim that they are externalist to an extent that would undermine biological psychiatry or the inclusive view of brain disorders. There is currently no convincing evidence for the claim that there are no qualitative or at least quantitative difference in the mental states (and correspondingly, the underlying brain states) which we label as disordered and those we label as healthy. The externalist case according to which there is no difference in the internal states of people suffering from mental disorder and those who have similar non-disordered internal states has been overstated.

Finally, we come to the practical implications of finding that mental disorders involve brain dysfunction and can therefore be counted as brain disorders on the inclusive view. Brain dysfunction is relevant to moral responsibility if and when it undermines the agent's capacities to understand the nature and morality of their action or their control over action. Whether this is the case needs to be decided at the psychological level, though brain findings can help to inform our judgements of whether, and to what extent, these capacities are impacted.

A further objection against the brain disorder label holds that this label affects the way people with a psychiatric diagnosis and their environment perceive them. If this is the case, agency may be impaired by the effect of the labels, irrespective of what effect the underlying condition itself might have. Empirical evidence on the effect of brain disorder labels is mixed, but does suggest some negative effects. Possible reasons for these effects are that people have the narrow model of brain disorders in mind, that they rely too heavily on paradigm cases, or that they are intuitive dualists. In as far as people are intuitive dualists who think of brain explanations for actions as undermining explanations in terms of reasoning processes, we should point out that this would pose problems for all agency, not just in the case of psychiatric disorders. Consequently, our response to negative labelling effects should be to counteract intuitive dualism, correct our view of brain disorders to a more inclusive one and broaden our diet of paradigm cases of brain disorder that we compare psychiatric illness to.

More generally, much of the resistance to the view that mental disorders are brain disorders rests on an understanding of the term 'brain disorder' that is both tendentious and not carefully thought through. This leads to unnecessary disagreements and polarization. It is my hope that this short book succeeds in shedding some light while reducing the heat, by showing what an inclusive account of brain disorders is actually committed to.

Bibliography

Aftab, Awais. 2020. "The False Binary between Biology and Behavior." *Philosophy, Psychiatry, & Psychology* 27 (3):317–319.

APA. 2013. *Diagnostic and Statistical Manual of Mental Disorder:DSM-5*. Fifth Edition. Arlington: American Psychiatric Association.

APA. 2020. "*What Is Schizophrenia*." Accessed 17.06.2021. https://www.psychiatry.org/patients-families/schizophrenia/what-is-schizophrenia.

Arpaly, Nomy. 2005. "How It Is not 'Just like Diabetes'. Mental Disorders and the Moral Psychologist." *Philosophical Issues* 15:282–298.

Associated Press. 2006. "Woman Not Guilty in Retrial in the Deaths of Her 5 Children." *New York Times*, 27.07.2006. Accessed 29.06.2021. https://www.nytimes.com/2006/07/27/us/27yates.html.

Banner, Natalie F. 2013. "Mental Disorders Are not Brain Disorders." *Journal of Evaluation in Clinical Practice* 19 (3):509–513. doi: 10.1111/jep.12048.

Bedi, Gillinder, Diana Martinez, Frances R. Levin, Sandra Comer, and Margaret Haney. 2017. "Addiction as a Brain Disease does not Promote Injustice." *Nature Human Behaviour* 1 (9):610–610. doi: 10.1038/s41562-017-0203-5.

Bell, V., S. Wilkinson, M. Greco, C. Hendrie, B. Mills, and Q. Deeley. 2020. "What Is the Functional/Organic Distinction Actually doing in Psychiatry and Neurology? [version 1; peer review: 3 approved]." *Wellcome Open Research* 5 (138). doi: 10.12688/wellcomeopenres.16022.1.

Berridge, Kent C. 2017. "Is Addiction a Brain Disease?" *Neuroethics* 10 (1):-29–33. doi: 10.1007/s12152-016-9286-3.

Bickle, John. 2010. "Has the Last Decade of Challenges to the Multiple Realization Argument Provided Aid and Comfort to Psychoneural Reductionists?" *Synthese* 177 (2):247–260. doi: 10.1007/s11229-010-9843-y.

Bird, Alexander, and Emma Tobin. 2022. "Natural Kinds." In *Stanford Encyclopedia of Philosophy*, edited by Edward Zalta. Accessed 28.02.2022. https://plato.stanford.edu/entries/natural-kinds/

Bolton, Derek. 2013. "Should Mental Disorders Be Regarded as Brain Disorders? 21st Century Mental Health Sciences and Implications for Research and Training." *World Psychiatry: Official Journal of the World Psychiatric Association (WPA)* 12 (1):24–25. doi: 10.1002/wps.20004.

Bolton, Derek, and Grant Gillett. 2019. *The Biopsychosocial Model of Health and Disease*. Cham: Palgrave MacMillan.

Boorse, Christopher. 1975. "On the Distinction between Disease and Illness." *Philosophy & Public Affairs* 5 (1):49–68.

Boorse, Christopher. 1977. "Health as a Theoretical Concept." *Philosophy of Science* 44 (4):542–573.

Borsboom, Denny, Angélique O. J. Cramer, and Annemarie Kalis. 2019. "Brain Disorders? Not Really: Why Network Structures Block Reductionism in Psychopathology Research." *Behavioral and Brain Sciences* 42 (e2):1–63. doi: 10.1017/S0140525X17002266.

Bortolotti, Lisa. 2020. "Doctors without 'Disorders'." *Aristotelian Society Supplementary Volume* 94 (1):163–184. doi: 10.1093/arisup/akaa006.

Bortolotti, Lisa, and Kengo Miyazono. 2015. "Recent Work on the Nature and Development of Delusions." *Philosophy Compass* 10 (9):636–645. doi: 10.1111/phc3.12249.

Boyd, Kenneth M. 2000. "Disease, Illness, Sickness, Health, Healing and Wholeness: Exploring Some Elusive Concepts." *Medical Humanities* 26 (1):9–17. doi: 10.1136/mh.26.1.9.

Broome, Matthew R., Lisa Bortolotti, and Matteo Mameli. 2010. "Moral Responsibility and Mental Illness: A Case Study." *Cambridge Quarterly of Healthcare Ethics* 19 (2):179–187. doi: 10.1017/S0963180109990442.

Burns, Jeffrey M., and Russell H. Swerdlow. 2003. "Right Orbitofrontal Tumor with Pedophilia Symptom and Constructional Apraxia Sign." *Archives of Neurology* 60 (3):437–440. doi: 10.1001/archneur.60.3.437.

Cooper, Rachel. 2007. *Psychiatry and Philosophy of Science*. Abingdon: Routledge.

Cooper, Rachel. 2013. "Natural Kinds." In *The Oxford Handbook of Philosophy and Psychiatry*, edited by K. W. M. Fulford, Martin Davies, George Graham, John Sadler, Giovanni Stanghellini and Tim Thornton, 950–965. Oxford: Oxford University Press.

Cooper, Rachel. 2020. "The Concept of Disorder Revisited: Robustly Value-Laden Despite Change." *Aristotelian Society Supplementary Volume* 94 (1):141–161. doi: 10.1093/arisup/akaa010.

Corlett, Philip. 2018. "Delusions and Prediction Error." In *Delusions in Context*, edited by Lisa Bortolotti, 35–66. Cham: Springer International Publishing.

Corrigan, P. W. 2007. "How Clinical Diagnosis Might Exacerbate the Stigma of Mental Illness." *Social Work* 52 (1):31–39. doi: 10.1093/sw/52.1.31.

Corrigan, Patrick W., and Amy C. Watson. 2004. "At Issue: Stop the Stigma: Call Mental Illness a Brain Disease." *Schizophrenia Bulletin* 30 (3):477–479. doi: 10.1093/oxfordjournals.schbul.a007095.

Cummins, Robert C. 1975. "Functional Analysis." *Journal of Philosophy* 72:741–764. doi: 10.1086/289488.

Davies, Will. 2016. "Externalist Psychiatry." *Analysis* 76 (3):290–296.

De Brigard, Felipe, Eric Mandelbaum, and David Ripley. 2008. "Responsibility and the Brain Sciences." *Ethical Theory and Moral Practice* 12 (5):511. doi: 10.1007/s10677-008-9143-5.

de Carvalho, M. R., M. Rozenthal, and A. E. Nardi. 2010. "The Fear Circuitry in Panic Disorder and Its Modulation by Cognitive-Behaviour Therapy Interventions." *The World Journal of Biological Psychiatry* 11 (2 Pt 2):188–198. doi: 10.1080/15622970903178176.

Department of Health. 2005. *Mental Capacity Act*. United Kingdom. Accessed 20.12.2021. https://www.legislation.gov.uk/ukpga/2005/9/contents.

Engel, George. 1977. "The Need for a New Medical Model: A Challenge for Biomedicine." *Science* 196:129–136.

Fagerberg, Harriet. 2022. "Why Mental Disorders Are not like Software Bugs." *Philosophy of Science* 1–42. doi: 10.1017/psa.2022.7

Farahany, Nita A. 2016. "Neuroscience and Behavioral Genetics in US Criminal Law: An Empirical Analysis." *Journal of Law and the Biosciences* 2 (3):485–509. doi: 10.1093/jlb/lsv059.

Fischer, John Martin, and Mark Ravizza. 1998. *Responsibility and Control: A Theory of Moral Responsibility*. Vol. 61. Cambridge, New York: Cambridge University Press.

Garson, Justin. 2011. "Selected Effects and Causal Role Functions in the Brain: The Case for an Etiological Approach to Neuroscience." *Biology & Philosophy* 26 (4):547–565. doi: 10.1007/s10539-011-9262-6.

Garson, Justin. 2019. *What Biological Functions Are and Why They Matter*. Cambridge: Cambridge University Press.

Glackin, Shane N. 2017. "Individualism and the Medical: What about Somatic Externalism?" *Analysis* 77 (2):287–293. doi: 10.1093/analys/anx073.

Goldberg, Anna E. 2020. "The (in)Significance of the Addiction Debate." *Neuroethics* 13 (3):311–324. doi: 10.1007/s12152-019-09424-5.

Graham, George. 2013a. *The Disordered Mind: An Introduction to Philosophy of Mind and Mental Illness*. Abingdon, New York: Routledge.

Graham, George. 2013b. "Ordering Disorder: Mental Disorder, Brain Disorder, and Therapeutic Intervention." In *The Oxford Handbook of Philosophy and Psychiatry*, edited by K. W. M. Fulford, Martin Davies, Richard G. T. Gipps, George Graham, John Sadler, Giovanni Stanghellini and Tim Thornton, 512–530. Oxford: Oxford University Press.

Graham, George. 2014. "Being a Mental Disorder." In *Classifying Psychopathology*, edited by Harold Kincaid and Jacqueline Sullivan, 123–143. Cambridge, MA: MIT Press.

Greene, Joshua, and Jonathan Cohen. 2011. "For the Law, Neuroscience Changes Nothing and Everything." In *The Oxford Handbook of Neuroethics*, edited by Judy Illes and Barbara Sahakian, 655–674. Oxford: Oxford University Press.

Hacking, Ian. 1995. *Rewriting the Soul: Multiple Personality and the Science of Memory*. Princeton, NJ: Princeton University Press.

Hacking, Ian. 2007. "Kinds of People: Moving Targets." In *Proceedings of the British Academy, Volume 151, 2006 Lectures*, 285–318.

Hacking, Ian. 2009. "Autistic Autobiography." *Philosophical Transactions of the Royal Society B: Biological Sciences* 364:1467–1473.

Hart, Carl L. 2017. "Viewing Addiction as a Brain Disease Promotes Social Injustice." *Nature Human Behaviour* 1:0055. doi: 10.1038/s41562-017-0055.

Heinrichs, Jan-Hendrik. 2019. *Neuroethik – Eine Einführung.* Stuttgart: J.B. Metzler.

Hirstein, William, Katrina Sifferd, and Tyler Fagan. 2018. *Responsible Brains: Neuroscience, Law and Human Culpability.* Cambridge, MA: MIT Press.

Holton, Richard, and Kent C. Berridge. 2013. "Addiction between Compulsion and Choice." In *Addiction and Self-Control, Perspectives from Philosophy, Psychology and Neuroscience*, edited by Neil Levy, 239–268. Oxford: Oxford University Press.

Horwitz, Allan, and Jerome C. Wakefield. 2007. *The Loss of Sadness: How Psychiatry Transformed Normal Sorrow into Depressive Disorder.* New York: Oxford University Press.

Hoyt, Crystal L., Jeni L. Burnette, and Lisa Auster-Gussman. 2014. "'Obesity Is a Disease': Examining the Self-Regulatory Impact of This Public-Health Message." *Psychological Science* 25 (4):997–1002. doi: 10.1177/0956797613516981.

Huda, Ahmed Samei. 2019. *The Medical Model in Mental Health: An Explanation and Evaluation.* New York: Oxford University Press.

Insel, T., B. Cuthbert, M. Garvey, R. Heinssen, D. S. Pine, K. Quinn, C. Sanislow, and P. Wang. 2010. "Research Domain Criteria (RDoC): Toward a New Classification Framework for Research on Mental Disorders." *The American Journal of Psychiatry* 167 (7):748–751. doi: 10.1176/appi.ajp.2010.09091379.

Insel, Thomas R., and Bruce N. Cuthbert. 2015. "Brain Disorders? Precisely." *Science* 348 (6234):499–500. doi: 10.1126/science.aab2358.

Jefferson, Anneli. 2014. "Mental Disorders, Brain Disorders and Values" *Frontiers in Psychology* 5:130. doi: 10.3389/fpsyg.2014.00130

Jefferson, Anneli. 2020a. "Confabulation, Rationalisation and Morality." *Topoi* 39 (1):219–227. doi: 10.1007/s11245-018-9608-7.

Jefferson, Anneli. 2020b. "What Does It Take to Be a Brain Disorder?" *Synthese* 197 (1):249–262. doi: 10.1007/s11229-018-1784-x.

Jefferson, Anneli. 2021. "On Mental Illness and Broken Brains." *Think* 20 (58):103–112. doi: 10.1017/S1477175621000099.

Jefferson, Anneli. 2022. "Brain Pathology and Moral Responsibility." In *Agency in Mental Disorder: Philosophical Dimensions*, edited by Joshua May and Matt King, 63–85. Oxford: Oxford University Press.

Jeppsson, Sofia. 2021. "Psychosis and Intelligibility." *Philosophy, Psychiatry, & Psychology* 28 (3):233–249.

Jurjako, Marko, and Luca Malatesti. 2020. "In What Sense Are Mental Disorders Brain Disorders? Explicating the Concept of Mental Disorder within RDoC." *Phenomenology and Mind* 18:182–198.

Kendler, K. S. 2005. "Toward a Philosophical Structure for Psychiatry." *American Journal of Psychiatry* 162 (3):433–440. doi: 10.1176/appi.ajp.162.3.433.

Kendler, K. S. 2012. "The Dappled Nature of Causes of Psychiatric Illness: Replacing the Organic-Functional/Hardware-Software Dichotomy with Empirically based Pluralism." *Molecular Psychiatry* 17 (4):377–388.

King, Matt, and Joshua May. 2018. "Moral Responsibility and Mental Illness: A Call for Nuance." *Neuroethics* 11 (1):11–22. doi: 10.1007/s12152-017-9345-4.

Kvaale, Erlend P., Nick Haslam, and William H. Gottdiener. 2013. "The 'Side Effects' of Medicalization: A Meta-Analytic Review of how Biogenetic Explanations Affect Stigma." *Clinical Psychology Review* 33 (6):782–794. doi: 10.1016/j.cpr.2013.06.002.

Kvaale, Erlend P., William H. Gottdiener, and Nick Haslam. 2013. "Biogenetic Explanations and Stigma: A Meta-Analytic Review of Associations among Laypeople." *Social Science & Medicine* 96:95–103. doi: 10.1016/j.socscimed.2013.07.017.

Lacasse, Jeffrey R., and Jonathan Leo. 2005. "Serotonin and Depression: A Disconnect between the Advertisements and the Scientific Literature." *PLoS Medicine* 2 (12):e392. doi: 10.1371/journal.pmed.0020392.

Leshner, A. I. 1997. "Addiction Is a Brain Disease, and It Matters." *Science* 278 (5335):45–47.

Levy, Neil. 2007. "The Responsibility of the Psychopath Revisited." *Philosophy, Psychiatry, and Psychology* 14 (2):129–138.

Lewis, Marc. 2017. "Addiction and the Brain: Development, Not Disease." *Neuroethics* 10 (1):7–18. doi: 10.1007/s12152-016-9293-4.

Lipska, Barbara. 2018. *The Neuroscientist who Lost Her Mind: A Memoir of Madness and Recovery.* London: Bantam Press.

Loughman, Amy, and Nick Haslam. 2018. "Neuroscientific Explanations and the Stigma of Mental Disorder: A Meta-Analytic Study." *Cognitive Research: Principles and Implications* 3 (1):43. doi: 10.1186/s41235-018-0136-1.

Maguire, Eleanor A., David G. Gadian, Ingrid S. Johnsrude, Catriona D. Good, John Ashburner, Richard S. J. Frackowiak, and Christopher D. Frith. 2000. "Navigation-Related Structural Change in the Hippocampi of Taxi Drivers." *Proceedings of the National Academy of Sciences* 97 (8):4398. doi: 10.1073/pnas.070039597.

Malla, Ashok, Ridha Joober, and Amparo Garcia. 2015. ""Mental Illness Is like Any Other Medical Illness"": A Critical Examination of the Statement and Its Impact on Patient Care and Society." *Journal of Psychiatry & Neuroscience: JPN* 40 (3):147–150. doi: 10.1503/jpn.150099.

Margolis, Eric, and Stephen Laurence. 2021. "Concepts." In *Stanford Encyclopedia of Philosophy*, edited by Edward Zalta. Accessed 12.12. 2021. https://plato.stanford.edu/archives/spr2021/entries/concepts/.

Maung, Hane Htut. 2019. "Dualism and Its Place in a Philosophical Structure for Psychiatry." *Medicine, Health Care and Philosophy* 22 (1):59–69. doi: 10.1007/s11019-018-9841-2.

Miresco, Marc J., and Laurence J. Kirmayer. 2006. "The Persistence of Mind-Brain Dualism in Psychiatric Reasoning about Clinical Scenarios." *American Journal of Psychiatry* 163 (5):913–918. doi: 10.1176/ajp.2006.163.5.913.

Mitchell, Sandra. 2012. *Unsimple Truths: Science, Complexity, and Policy.* Chicago, IL: Chicago University Press.

Moncrieff, Joanna. 2020. """It Was the Brain Tumor That Done It!"": Szasz and Wittgenstein on the Importance of Distinguishing Disease from Behavior and Implications for the Nature of Mental Disorder." *Philosophy, Psychiatry, & Psychology* 27 (2):169–181.

Morse, Stephen J. 2008. "Psychopathy and Criminal Responsibility." *Neuroethics* 1 (3):205–212

Morse, Stephen. 2011a. "Avoiding Irrational NeuroLaw Exuberance: A Plea for Neuromodesty." *Mercer Law Review* 62:837–859.

Morse, Stephen. 2011b. "Lost in Translation? An Essay on Law and Neuroscience." In *Law and Neuroscience: Current Legal Issues Volume 13*, edited by Michael Freeman, 529–562. Oxford: Oxford University Press.

Morse, Stephen J. 2017. "Neuroethics: Neurolaw." In *Oxford Handbooks Online*. https://www.oxfordhandbooks.com/view/10.1093/oxfordhb/9780199935314. 001.0001/oxfordhb-9780199935314-e-45

Mottron, Laurent. 2011. "The Power of Autism." *Nature* 479:33–35.

NHS. 2020. "*Trombophilia.*" Accessed 23.06.2021. https://www.nhs.uk/conditions/thrombophilia/.

NIDA. 2020. "*Drugs and the Brain.*". Accessed 05.07.2021. https://www.drugabuse.gov/publications/drugs-brains-behavior-science-addiction/drugs-brain.

NIMH. "About RDoC." Accessed 22.06.2021. https://www.nimh.nih.gov/research/research-funded-by-nimh/rdoc/about-rdoc.shtml.

Nord, Camilla. 2021. "Mental Disorders Are Brain Disorders – Here's why this Matters." *Psyche.* Accessed 14.09.2021. https://psyche.co/ideas/mental-disorders-are-brain-disorders-heres-why-that-matters.

Nord, Camilla L., D. Chamith Halahakoon, Tarun Limbachya, Caroline Charpentier, Níall Lally, Vincent Walsh, Judy Leibowitz, Stephen Pilling, and Jonathan P. Roiser. 2019. "Neural Predictors of Treatment Response to Brain Stimulation and Psychological Therapy in Depression: A Double-Blind Randomized Controlled Trial." *Neuropsychopharmacology* 44 (9):1613–1622. doi: 10.1038/s41386-019-0401-0.

Papineau, David. 1994. "Mental Disorder, Illness and Biological Disfunction." *Royal Institute of Philosophy Supplements* 37:73–82. doi: 10.1017/S135824610000998X.

Parcesepe, A. M., and L. J. Cabassa. 2013. "Public Stigma of Mental Illness in the United States: A Systematic Literature Review." *Administration and Policy in Mental Health and Mental Health Services Research* 40 (5):384–399. doi: 10.1007/s10488-012-0430-z.

Pernu, Tuomas K. 2019. "Elimination, not Reduction: Lessons from the Research Domain Criteria (RDoC) and Multiple Realisation." *Behavioral and Brain Sciences* 42 (e22):32–33.

Pessoa, Luiz. 2019. "Brain Networks for Emotion and Cognition: Implications and Tools for Understanding Mental Disorders and Pathophysiology." *Behavioral and Brain Sciences* 42 (e23):33–35. doi: 10.1017/S0140525X18001140.

Pickard, Hanna. 2018. "Mental Disorders are Real, Diagnosis or Not." *Institute of Art and Ideas*, 65. Accessed 20.12.2021. https://iai.tv/articles/why-do-we-need-a-diagnosis-to-see-mental-disorders-as-real-auid-1067.

Pompanin, Sara, Nela Jelcic, Diego Cecchin, and Annachiara Cagnin. 2014. "Impulse Control Disorders in Frontotemporal Dementia: Spectrum of Symptoms and Response to Treatment." *General Hospital Psychiatry* 36 (6):760.e5–760.e7. doi: 10.1016/j.genhosppsych.2014.06.005.

Putnam, Hilary. 1975. "The Meaning of 'Meaning'." *Minnesota Studies in the Philosophy of Science* 7:131–193.

Radden, Jennifer. 2018. "Rethinking Disease in Psychiatry: Disease Models and the Medical Imaginary." *Journal of Evaluation in Clinical Practice* 24 (5):1087–1092. doi: 10.1111/jep.12982.

Roache, Rebecca. 2020. "The Biopsychosocial Model in Psychiatry: Engel and Beyond." In *Psychiatry Reborn: Biopsychosocial Psychiatry in Modern Medicine*, edited by Julian Savulescu, Rebecca Roache and Will Davies, 6–22. New York: Oxford University Press.

Roberts, Tom, Joel Krueger, and Shane Glackin. 2019. "Psychiatry beyond the Brain: Externalism, Mental Health, and Autistic Spectrum Disorder." *Philosophy, Psychiatry, & Psychology* 26 (3):51–68. doi: doi:10.1353/ppp.2019.0030.

Roiser, Jonathan P., Rebecca Elliott, and Barbara J. Sahakian. 2012. "Cognitive Mechanisms of Treatment in Depression." *Neuropsychopharmacology* 37 (1):117–136. doi: 10.1038/npp.2011.183.

Rose, Beth. 2017. "'What's Mum Got to Be Depressed About?'." *BBC News*, 23.02.2017. https://www.bbc.co.uk/news/disability-38929093.

Satel, Sally, and Scott Lilienfeld. 2017. "Calling It 'Brain Disease' Makes Addiction Harder to Treat. " *Boston Globe*. https://www.bostonglobe.com/ideas/2017/06/22/calling-brain-disease-makes-addiction-harder-treat/ehaJs5ZYIXpPottG89KOGK/story.html.

Schramme, Thomas. 2010. "Can We Define Mental Disorder by Using the Criterion of Mental Dysfunction?" *Theoretical Medicine and Bioethics* 31 (1):35–47. doi: 10.1007/s11017-010-9136-y.

Schramme, Thomas. 2013. "On the Autonomy of the Concept of Disease in Psychiatry." *Frontiers in Psychology* 4 (457). doi: 10.3389/fpsyg.2013.00457.

Sinnott-Armstrong, Walter, Adina Roskies, Teneille Brown, and Emily Murphy. 2008. "Brain Images as Legal Evidence." *Episteme* 5 (3):359–373. doi: 10.3366/E1742360008000452.

Szasz, Thomas. 1960. "The Myth of Mental Illness." *American Psychologist* 15:113–118.

Szasz, Thomas. 2011. "The Myth of Mental Illness: 50 Years Later." *The Psychiatrist* 35 (5):179–182. doi: 10.1192/pb.bp.110.031310.

Vincent, Nicole A. 2008. "Responsibility, Dysfunction and Capacity." *Neuroethics* 1 (3):199–204. doi: 10.1007/s12152-008-9022-8.

Wakefield, Jerome C. 1992a. "The Concept of Mental Disorder. On the Boundary between Biological Facts and Social Values." *American Psychologist* 47 (3):373–388.

Wakefield, Jerome C. 1992b. "Disorder as Harmful Dysfunction – A Conceptual Critique of DSM III-R's Definition of Mental Disorder." *Psychological Review* 99 (2):232–247.

Wakefield, Jerome C. 2000. "Spandrels, Vestigial Organs, and Such: Reply to Murphy and Woolfolk's '"The Harmful Dysfunction Analysis of Mental Disorder'"." *Philosophy, Psychiatry, and Psychology* 7 (4):253–269.

Wakefield, Jerome 2017a. "Addiction and the Concept of Disorder, Part 2: Is every Mental Disorder a Brain Disorder?" *Neuroethics* 1–13. doi: 10.1007/s12152-016-9301-8.

Wakefield, Jerome C. 2017b. "Addiction and the Concept of Disorder, Part 1: Why Addiction is a Medical Disorder." *Neuroethics* 10 (1):39–53. doi: 10.1007/s12152-016-9300-9.

Walter, Henrik. 2013. "The Third Wave of Biological Psychiatry." *Frontiers in Psychology* 4 (582). doi: 10.3389/fpsyg.2013.00582.

Watson, Jo, ed. 2019. *Drop the Disorder.* London: PCCS Books.

Wilkinson, G. 1986. "Political Dissent and '"Sluggish'" Schizophrenia in the Soviet Union." *British Medical Journal (Clinical Research ed.)* 293 (6548):641–642. doi: 10.1136/bmj.293.6548.641.

Yehuda, Rachel, Charles W. Hoge, Alexander C. McFarlane, Eric Vermetten, Ruth A. Lanius, Caroline M. Nievergelt, Stevan E. Hobfoll, Karestan C. Koenen, Thomas C. Neylan, and Steven E. Hyman. 2015. "Post-Traumatic Stress Disorder." *Nature Reviews Disease Primers* 1 (1):15057. doi: 10.1038/nrdp.2015.57.

Zimmerman, Mark, William Ellison, Diane Young, Iwona Chelminski, and Kristy Dalrymple. 2015. "How Many Different Ways Do Patients Meet the Diagnostic Criteria for Major Depressive Disorder?" *Comprehensive Psychiatry* 56:29–34. doi: 10.1016/j.comppsych.2014.09.007.

Index

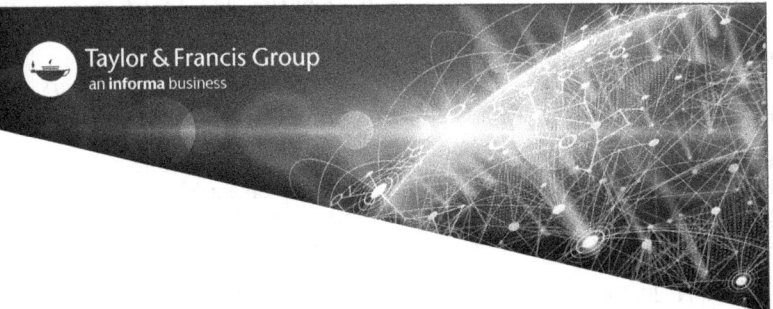
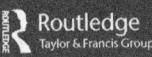
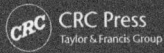